BEHIND CLOSED DOORS

BEHIND
CLOSED DOORS

Uncovering the Practices Harming
Our Children's Health
...and What We CAN *Do About It*

JOANNE STANTON & CHRISTINE O'DONNELL

NEW YORK

NASHVILLE • MELBOURNE • VANCOUVER

BEHIND CLOSED DOORS

Uncovering the Practices Harming Our
Children's Health and What We CAN Do About It

© 2018 JOANNE STANTON & CHRISTINE O'DONNELL

Published in New York, New York, by Morgan James Publishing. Morgan James is a trademark of Morgan James, LLC. www.MorganJamesPublishing.com

The Morgan James Speakers Group can bring authors to your live event. For more information or to book an event visit The Morgan James Speakers Group at www.TheMorganJamesSpeakersGroup.com.

ISBN 978-1-68350-575-4 paperback
ISBN 978-1-68350-576-1 eBook
Library of Congress Control Number: 2017907211

Cover Design by:
Nika Tchaikovskaya with
Rachel Lopez, www.r2cdesign.com

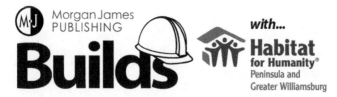

In an effort to support local communities, raise awareness and funds, Morgan James Publishing donates a percentage of all book sales for the life of each book to Habitat for Humanity Peninsula and Greater Williamsburg.

Get involved today! Visit
www.MorganJamesBuilds.com

Believe nothing, no matter where you read it,
or who said it, no matter if I have said it,
unless it agrees with your own reason
and your own common sense.

—commonly attributed to Buddha

*This book is dedicated to our children
Patrick, Colin, Brendan, Erin, James, Conor, and Kaleigh;
and to all the precious children of this world.*

*May your future be filled with health, joy,
abundance, and unlimited possibilities.*

TABLE OF CONTENTS

ACKNOWLEDGMENTS

First and foremost, to our husbands Marty and John, your unwavering support in every way has enabled this book to come to fruition. Your faith in us and your belief in the importance of the information we share truly shows your love and commitment not only to our own children but to all children. Our deepest thanks and gratitude for standing beside us the entire way. And to our own children, thanks for your patience and understanding during this eight-year endeavor that often took time away from you. We hope it has taught you to stand up for what you believe in.

Words cannot express our heartfelt appreciation to all of our friends and family who provided support, encouragement, and love along the way. There are too many of you to list. You know who you are—*thank you* from the bottom of our hearts. Your simple words of encouragement and interest in our project kept us going and validated the vital information we wanted to share. A special acknowledgment goes out to the many in this group that were also brave enough to read early portions of the manuscript and give us feedback. Your efforts helped provide early vision for the book and shaped it into what it is today.

We are forever indebted and deeply thankful to Stephen Singular, *New York Times* best-selling author, who reviewed our manuscript and encouraged us to tell our stories and the stories of the many mothers we spoke to along the way. This book would not have been as impactful if we had not made it so personal. Thank you for your vision and guidance in sharing our stories and for being so confident that our manuscript was of value and would be well received.

A special thanks to Dr. Scott Shannon, who provided us with expert medical review of the entire manuscript. Our sincere gratitude for squeezing us into your busy schedule and for the positive feedback you provided. It is our sincere hope that your holistic and integrative approach to children's health one day becomes the norm.

Our heartfelt gratitude goes out to Jim Turner, one of our country's leading attorneys, whose lifework has been dedicated to protecting consumers. Thank you for taking the time out of your very busy practice to provide legal review of the manuscript and for wholeheartedly believing in the messages it contained. Thanks also go out to our copyright lawyer Joe Maenner; your legal guidance and calm reassurance during this whole process was a gift.

Additionally, we would like to acknowledge the many other invaluable early manuscript reviews provided by those working in specific content areas: Angela Gerolamo, PhD; Sarah Bauerle Bass, PhD; Suzanne Cardie, CRNP; Bill Walker; Theresa Wrangham; and Sara Jennings. Thank you all for sharing your professional insights and essential feedback.

To our wonderfully talented editor Amanda Rooker, thank you from the bottom of our hearts for believing in us and providing us with expert guidance. Your editorial skills and knowledge of the industry kept us sailing on a steady path to publishing. Your sincere interest in the messages contained within the book meant more to us than you will ever know.

To the brilliant duo of Nika Tchaikovskaya (artist) and Natalie Chaykina (graphic designer). We were blessed to have found the both of you! Thank you for working so patiently with us over the years and for always believing in the importance of this work. Your beautiful artwork and creativity helped weave heart, love, and light into every page of the book. You managed to lighten some heavy topics and helped us create a book that was reader friendly. Thank you for sticking with us through the entire project. You both have hearts of gold.

A special thank you to Mark Van der Gaag for your support and encouragement when the book was just an idea. Your unwavering belief that awakening the mothers would change the world kept us moving forward.

We are also forever grateful to the many mothers we met along the way who candidly shared conversations and personal stories with us concerning their own children's health. Your struggles, strength, and victories fueled us to continue working to bring these vital issues to the forefront of conversations.

A huge thank you to the many grassroots consumer advocacy organizations that shared our vision of health and vitality for children and our planet. Many of you provided us with information or graphics to use in the book and offered a wealth of information to present our readers with in the Resource Guide, both in the book and online at www.behindcloseddoorsthebook.com. Thank you for encouraging us to press on to get this book finalized and in the hands of readers.

Our sincere appreciation also goes out to those working at government agencies such as the FDA, CDC, USDA, and EPA who patiently answered a barrage of our questions and inquiries while doing research.

And finally, there is one special person without whom this book could not have been completed: Mary Lou Cardie. Your faith in this project never wavered even when ours sometimes did. Words cannot express the gratitude we hold in our hearts for all your contributions. Thank you for sharing your inspiring personal story with us so others could benefit. We appreciate the time and talents you dedicated to the project over the years. From continually reviewing and providing excellent feedback on every single draft of the manuscript we sent your way to organizing and formatting hundreds of citations, this book could not have been birthed without you.

IMPORTANT NOTES TO READERS

This book received expert medical review by Scott M. Shannon, MD, who is board certified in child and adolescent psychiatry and integrative holistic medicine. It also received additional scientific and medical reviews that were content specific. Dr. Shannon is Assistant Clinical Professor of Psychiatry at the University of Colorado and past president of the American Board of Integrative Holistic Medicine. He teaches healthcare professionals around the world how to approach children's health and well-being holistically.

The information presented in this book is not intended as medical advice, and its contents should not be considered a substitute for professional medical treatment or diagnosis. This book is based upon the opinions of the respective authors. Its content is intended as a sharing of knowledge and information from the research and personal experiences of the authors. The authors encourage you to make your own healthcare decisions based upon your own research and in partnership with a qualified healthcare professional.

WHAT'S HAPPENING TO OUR CHILDREN'S HEALTH?

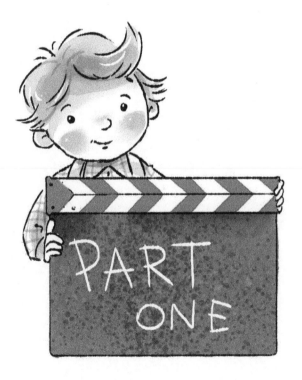

Chapter 1

AN URGENT MESSAGE

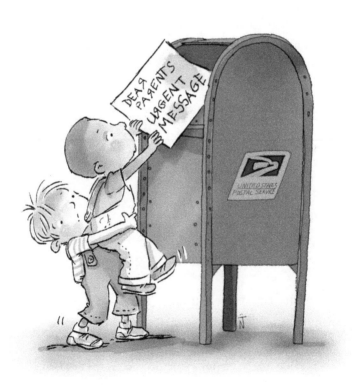

When sleeping women wake, mountains move.
—Chinese Proverb

A s busy moms, it takes our full energy and focus just to keep up with our normal daily schedule: diapers, feeding, kids' activities, school and homework, sports and music practices—not to mention our own careers, homes, and significant relationships. It often takes a major shock to our system to get us to pay attention to anything outside the hectic world we live in. For both of us, that shock came the day we each separately received a serious health diagnosis for our small children. Our protective instincts kicked in and set us on a path to find answers. We soon found out we weren't alone in our experience or our questioning.

Chronic disease and disability in U.S. children are at an all-time high, and we as mothers simply want to know, why? What is happening to our children? Was it always like this? What is causing it? And most importantly, what can we do about it?

These questions continued to tug at our heart as we heard about more and more children in our families and neighborhoods with autism, food allergies, learning disabilities, and mental health disorders. It was our simple conversations with other moms at bus stops, grocery stores, and sports fields that highlighted the reality of the growing problem, the deep impact it was having on families, and the need to do something about it.

We invite you to share our journey from the very beginning. Below are our personal stories that launched our quest to find answers.

Flight or Fight: Joanne's Story

In the summer of 1991, I (Joanne) had three children: Patrick was six and getting ready to start first grade, Colin was three, and Brendan was just four months old. Patrick began having severe migraines in the mornings, along with bouts of vomiting and problems maintaining his balance. As he got progressively worse, a brain MRI was scheduled. The day before the procedure our family took a walk together. Patrick could barely keep his feet on the sidewalk, drifting off into the grass on either side as we walked. I hoped he had an inner ear infection or another simple explanation for his balance problems. One of my greatest passions was coaching high school field hockey, and the morning of Patrick's MRI, I planned out my team's evening practice—not knowing that my life as a coach and as a mother was about to change forever.

My husband, Marty, and I took Patrick to the MRI, a procedure that would last an extremely long forty-five minutes. Thankfully, we were allowed in the MRI room with him. As he underwent what can be a very scary and claustrophobic experience, Patrick was brave, especially for a small child. A female technician behind a glass window spoke to him through a microphone and watched a computer screen showing the results of the exam in real time. Within the first few minutes, it was clear that something was wrong. Others soon joined her and looked concerned as they pointed at the screen and talked, but we could hear nothing. One picked up the phone to make a call and the remaining thirty minutes of the MRI were painfully slow as we feared what news may be coming.

When the MRI was finished, Patrick was offered an overabundance of treats—lollipops, stickers, and small toys. We were asked to stay there as they developed the film of the procedure, and several minutes later, a nurse instructed us to take the film to Patrick's doctor immediately. They'd already called our physician and he knew we were on our way. We dropped Patrick off at home with my mother, who was watching his two younger brothers. I'll never forget the moment we stepped foot inside our doctor's office. I knew several of the women who worked there and each one noticeably avoided me, glancing away or getting up to leave as I approached the front desk.

The doctor was only about thirty years old and visibly upset by what he had to do next.

"There's no easy way to tell you this," he said. "Patrick has a tumor about the size of a golf ball in the back of his brain. The brain tumor is causing his migraines and balance problems. It is also blocking some of the spinal fluid in the brain, and that's creating immense pressure that could result in an aneurysm. You've got to get to the hospital now. They're waiting for you."

They say that in a crisis some people fall apart, while others rise up. It really is fight or flight. After hearing those devastating words, a calm came over me and I sat up and paid close attention. I was ready for the fight.

"What hospital?" I asked. "What floor? What's the plan once we get him there?"

We drove home in utter shock and then flew into action. My husband packed some clothes and I went to find Patrick. How could I explain this to him? I simply stated the truth.

"The pictures they took of your head showed something growing in there that shouldn't be there. It's causing your headaches, your throwing up, and your balance problems. This is good news because we now know what's wrong and we can begin to take care of it."

At the hospital, we were told that there was so much swelling in the brain that immediate surgery was too dangerous. They put Patrick on steroids for three days to bring this down, in preparation for the operation.

The night before the surgery, I couldn't sleep. I left Patrick's hospital room at Children's Hospital of Philadelphia (CHOP) and went down the hall to the children's playroom. Sitting alone on the floor in the dark, I cried hard for the first time since learning about the tumor. I sobbed for hours. I prayed and prayed as I cried. I also got angry and questioned why this had happened to my six-year-old son. Why couldn't I have a brain tumor instead? And then, at one of the lowest points in my life, something strange happened, an experience I'd never had before and haven't had since: I physically "felt" a huge hug wash over me. This very real and very warm embrace lasted for just a few seconds. In that moment I knew I wasn't alone and this filled me with peace. I knew that somehow our family would get through this.

The next morning Patrick went into surgery at CHOP. An Amish family was there for the same reason, as were other families from all over the East Coast. The message was obvious: cancer can strike anyone and people everywhere have to deal with the consequences. I was so thankful that I lived near a major city, an hour's drive to one of the best pediatric hospitals in the world. When the operation was over, the doctor came out and told us that everything had gone well.

"The tumor practically fell out in my hand," he said. "I am confident that I got it all, but we still need to send it off for a biopsy. I've seen a lot of these and my instinct is that we are dealing with cancer." The results would later confirm that he was right.

Within the hour, they'd wheeled Patrick out of the operating room and he was headed to the ICU. He was attached to a variety of monitoring devices and had his entire head wrapped up. The nurse smiled and handed me a cup.

"You can show Patrick this when he wakes up," she told me. "He lost his first tooth while we were in there. Maybe you can put it under his pillow tonight."

While Patrick was in the ICU, we learned that our four-month-old son, Brendan, had been diagnosed with severe asthma. He was having a spate of respiratory illnesses and infections. Before his second birthday, Brendan would be in the hospital on at least a dozen occasions, and both Brendan and Patrick were at times hospitalized simultaneously.

Following Patrick's surgery, he couldn't walk. So many of his neck muscles had been cut through that he also struggled to turn his head to say no or yes. He started physical therapy and we met with his doctor to lay out a two-year treatment plan that included intensive radiation treatment to his head and spine, as well as three different types of chemotherapy.

Immediately following his surgery and initial diagnosis, a doctor pummeled my husband and me with pointed questions: Where did we live? Where did we work? Did we live near a farm? Had we ever used or been around pesticides? Where did each of us grow up? Until now, I hadn't thought about any of these things, but I was now jolted into learning everything I could.

I began doing research and discovered that many childhood cancers, especially brain tumors and leukemias, have strong links to environmental causes. I also learned that a few other children from the small town where we were living had also been recently diagnosed with cancerous brain tumors. Could my son's illness be related to an environmental factor, like a nearby nuclear power plant, or a local EPA Superfund site? Or could it be the result of earlier environmental exposures during my pregnancy? I'd begun to question everything. Through my research, I built a knowledge base about pediatric brain tumors, environmental health, learning disabilities, and the devastating effects that chemotherapy and radiation can have on a child's body and developing brain.

Although it was painful to watch my small son endure chemo, radiation, and the countless side effects associated with initial treatment, it didn't begin to compare to the slow and sometimes cruel long-term effects that still continue to surface more than twenty years later. Watching a bright and vibrant child slowly fade into a mildly disabled adult was far more heartbreaking than the two years we spent battling the disease. Thankfully, less toxic therapies are now used to treat children with cancer and quality-of-life outcomes have improved.

My son's brain tumor set me on a course of self-education that's unfolded over the past twenty-five years, all in an effort to raise awareness about the many causes and effects of cancer. I now realize that so much needless suffering in our country could be prevented through stronger regulations governing environmental pollutants and consumer products containing chemicals known or suspected to cause cancer. Our best hope is not in treatments, but in preventing this devastating disease from ever happening.

During Patrick's battle with cancer, his two younger brothers also had their share of medical problems. These experiences gave me a unique perspective into other health challenges, including severe asthma, speech delays, mild learning disabilities, gastrointestinal problems, hearing impairments, and a documented serious vaccine reaction.

An Alternative Way: Christine's Story

Around the turn of the new millennium, I (Christine) had three children: Erin was six, James was five, and Conor was two. Later that year, I gave birth to my fourth child. When I heard my husband John exclaim, "It's a girl!" I remember how thrilled I was to know Erin now had a sister. Kaleigh was born vibrant and healthy. My life was busy with four little ones at home and a husband who traveled a lot for work. Despite occasional exhaustion, at the end of each day I felt that my life was perfect.

At about nine months of age, and just days after she'd received her scheduled vaccinations, I began noticing significant changes in Kaleigh. Within two weeks, she'd developed a slew of mysterious symptoms that included hives, a body rash, a diaper rash, an ear infection, bouts of gastrointestinal problems, fits of unexplained crying, and severe eczema on her face to the point that it bled. Back and forth we went to the doctors for the next several months. As these conditions persisted, I grew weary from wanting answers. My pediatrician had no solutions but was able to provide medications to help control her many symptoms. I had three other children, so I knew that it was far from normal for an infant to be chronically ill. I was increasingly overwhelmed and scared for my daughter.

Our pediatrician finally referred us to an allergist who diagnosed Kaleigh with asthma, as well as life-threatening peanut and seafood allergies. She also proved to be allergic to bananas, wheat, eggs, and dairy. Although somewhat relieved that I now had some useful information, I questioned why a toddler would be allergic to so many different foods and was terrified by the thought that my daughter could possibly die if she came into contact with peanuts or seafood. I was grateful to have an EpiPen, an epinephrine autoinjector to deal with her condition, but how could I protect her from exposures?

For the next six weeks we used medications to control her asthma and made extensive changes in her diet. Although I was very thankful that a few of Kaleigh's symptoms improved slightly, many of her problems persisted. The list of her medications was growing, and I even received a letter from the allergist asking if we would be interested in having Kaleigh partake in a clinical drug trial for asthma. This was my breaking point. Everything in my gut told me that I needed to find an alternative way of dealing with Kaleigh' symptoms, so I sought out a medical doctor with a background in both environmental medicine and homeopathy. He ordered extensive testing to see if he could get to the root of her problems.

A few days before Thanksgiving, as we were preparing for a trip to John's family in Connecticut, Kaleigh's test results came back from our new doctor. The biochemical analysis showed a multitude of toxins wreaking havoc in her tiny eighteen-month-old body. The report, similar to a toxicology report, also warned us of what other illnesses and disabilities could potentially lay ahead if we didn't reduce Kaleigh's high levels of heavy metals and toxins. I was overwhelmed. How could a toddler's body become so toxic? Where were all these toxins coming from? How could I get rid of them and avoid them in the future? Mercury, aluminum, cadmium, arsenic, antimony . . . the list went on and on. As I read the report, my search for truth began. What I uncovered bewildered me. Why was a toxic chemical like antimony in baby products? Why was mercury used in infant vaccinations? Why was cadmium in children's toys?

Protectors of Our Children

Inevitably, both of our experiences forced us to take a closer look at many of our everyday practices. In doing our research we began to realize just how naïve and unaware we really were. Many consumer products that we had assumed to be completely safe for our children simply were not, and as mothers this was difficult to discover. We started to ask ourselves a litany of questions:

- What are all those chemical ingredients in the food we're serving our families?
- Are there any long-term effects from the daily medications our children take?
- Are the soaps, sunblock, and diapers we use on our children's bodies tested and safe?
- Why are so many of the same products for sale in the United States banned in other countries?
- Have we been blindly accepting another's assessment of what is safe and appropriate for our children?

Like most mothers, the more we discovered the answers to these questions, the more we started to realize that, in some ways, we had failed to protect our children.

Sadly, we came to understand that in today's world, we are ultimately the ones responsible for safeguarding our children against an ever-growing list of potential toxins. But should we have to be? It is our government's job to protect our children from harmful consumer products. This is the very purpose of our political system and chemical regulations. We shouldn't have to read every label to see if a product on a store shelf is safe or harmful. But until laws change, this is our reality.

All of this questioning on behalf of our children led to unearthing more and more critical consumer information. For instance, did you know that mercury, one of the most highly toxic chemicals and extremely harmful to children's brains, is present in our new energy-efficient CFL lightbulbs and in silver "amalgam" dental fillings? Did you know that ingredients like aluminum, formaldehyde,

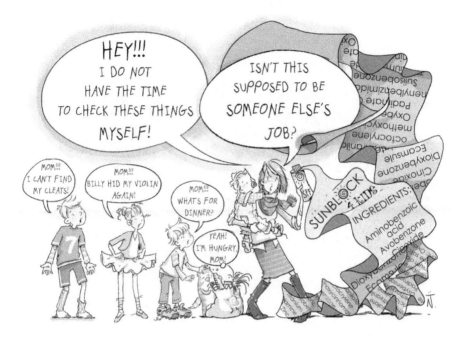

and thimerosal, all known to be toxic to the brain, are present in some childhood vaccinations? Did you know that 94 percent of the soy and 93 percent of the corn in the U.S. food system have been genetically modified from their natural form and that we've been eating these and other genetically modified food products since the early 1990s?

Many of us don't know these things unless we work in related industries, and even then many are still in the dark. We began to explore these practices and many more so we could understand what was happening to our children's health.

We took a simple, common-sense approach. It seemed as though many children's health disorders were on the rise over the past few decades. So we decided to compare U.S. children's health statistics from today to those from just twenty to thirty years ago. Would it validate our concerns? We then asked, what has changed in many of our nation's key industries over the same time period? Could some of our everyday practices (such as the food we eat) be contributing factors to our children's health problems? As we will continue to demonstrate over and over, the proof lies in the statistics. Based on our research and our personal experiences with our own children, we believe that

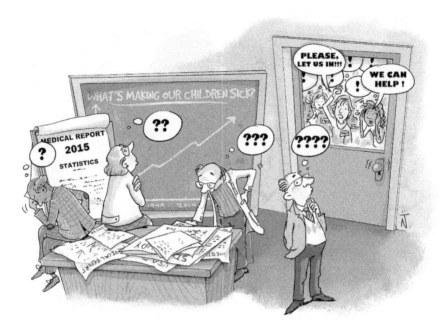

the increases in many children's health disorders are the collective effects of changed practices within our food industry, environment, medical protocols, and most importantly our laws.

It goes without saying that we are extremely thankful to have the technology and advancements these industries have contributed to our society. However, in an effort to make improvements, provide conveniences, and in some instances even attempt to improve the health of our children and the laws of our nation, did we create practices that have grown out of balance as a result?

We will share with you all we have learned and invite you to draw your own conclusions to the many questions we will continually raise throughout this book. How have industry practices changed over the past few decades? Do these changes serve the interests of our children or the interest of the industry? Do these practices play a part in the rise of many of our children's health problems? And if so, what can we do about it?

Naturally, each separate industry will defend itself by saying, "It is not us; we are not responsible." However, what they may fail to see is that it is not just one industry alone. It is the sum of the parts that together equals the whole. We will show you how a little bit of this and a little bit of that can quickly add up. The combined and cumulative effects of food, chemicals, and even pharmaceuticals can take a toll on our children's developing bodies.

Now, more than ever, we are called to be protectors of our children. A mother can and will, without fail, safeguard her child—for her love is strong and her protection fierce. Once a mother's heart is awakened to the truth of what is playing out behind closed doors regarding her children, she will not be silenced. She will not be stopped.

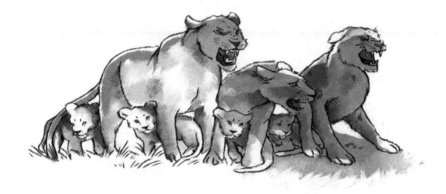

 This icon will let you know that more information can be found in the **Resource Guide**, located in Part 3 of this book. The Resource Guide provides supplemental information on many of the topics we will explore together. It also includes helpful links to the websites of various organizations and federal agencies offering additional tools and support to help you navigate your family to better health.

Also, we'll be continually updating this Resource Guide online as we become aware of more information. Go to www.behindcloseddoorsthebook.com to download a free electronic version of the Resource Guide, and sign up to receive updated versions as soon as they're released.

Chapter 2

THE UNDERLYING ISSUES

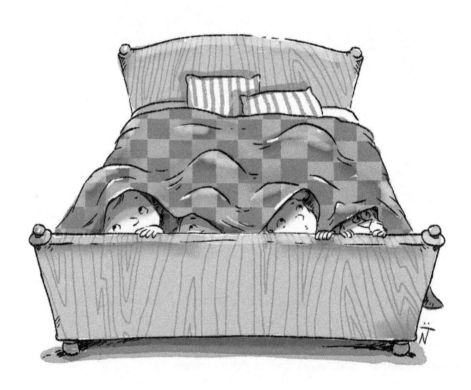

Our lives begin to end the day we become silent
about the things that matter.
—Martin Luther King Jr.

T oday, one in every fifty children develops an autism-related disorder. The number of children on psychiatric medications is soaring. In recent years, the number of children with diabetes, asthma, and food allergies has more than doubled. And right here in the United States, we have more infants die during the first year of life than in fifty-six other countries in the world. What has compromised our children's immune system so drastically that for the first time in U.S. history, many of today's children are not expected to live as healthy or as long as their parents? How in the United States of America can this be true?

Let's start with the basics. When we harm the environment, we ultimately harm ourselves. Spraying apple orchards with toxic pesticides not only contaminates the apples and the child who may eat the apple, but the surrounding land and waterways, as well as the plants and animals inhabiting both. One small action affects the entire ecosystem: toxic practices yield toxic bodies. It's that simple, and it's really just common sense. The detrimental effects of any environmental damage will be seen first in the health and well-being of our infants and children because their small bodies are more susceptible. Infants and children absorb and retain higher levels of certain contaminants because their bodies cannot detoxify as quickly as adults.

In the United States we're emitting some of the highest levels of toxins in the world, producing four billion pounds of industrial pollution a year. Should it be any surprise that we're seeing the effects of this on our health? Or that breast milk from nursing mothers contains toxins? Why have we allowed dangerous chemicals to flourish in all types of consumer goods? Where is the responsibility of our government agencies charged with protecting our food, environment, consumer goods, and most importantly our children? We will not be able to move forward with any meaningful reform unless we have the courage to examine how we got here.

What Started It All?

> *We don't have to engage in grand, heroic actions to*
> *participate in the process of change. Small acts, when*
> *multiplied by millions of people, can transform the world.*
> —Howard Zinn

After World War II, American industry exploded. Technological advancements supported the creation of products to make our everyday living simpler. Businesses started creating the "convenience factor" in all types of consumer products including food, medicine, and general goods. The end result of many of these conveniences has been a seriously polluted environment, and in turn, seriously polluted human bodies. Most of us realize that chemical pollutants can end up in our air, water, and soil, but many are surprised to learn that they ultimately end up in our bodies (Kaleigh's story is a testament to this).

High levels of toxins and heavy metals have been found not only in the blood and urine of U.S. children, but in the umbilical cord blood of newborn babies as well. This is proof positive that dangerous substances contained in or produced by many of our modern conveniences are getting into our bodies and the bodies of our children. Where are these toxins coming from? And how can we reduce what our children are being exposed to?

Since around 1950, we've successfully introduced into our world more than 80,000 synthetic chemicals and have only tested the effects of about 200 of these on humans. Many were never intended for human consumption, but due to the symbiotic relationship we have with the earth we're absorbing them into our bodies. For example, chemical-laden products we discard as trash are burned in incinerators, which can result in the carcinogen dioxin being released into the air that our children, pets, and wildlife breathe.

Other chemicals are intentionally manufactured into our food, medicine, and consumer goods for our own convenience and sometimes even our own protection. While manufacturers are aware that their products will be consumed by, or come in contact with, humans, their health effects were not always taken into consideration during the planning process. As a result, we have flame-retardant chemicals present in many infant and baby products that are now linked to cancer, birth defects, infertility, and neurological disorders. Many children's toys contain phthalates, a class of chemicals linked to reproductive issues and early onset puberty. We have butylated hydroxytoluene (BHT), a chemical preservative linked to behavioral problems, infertility, a weakened immune system, and other health issues, in many of our food products, like breakfast cereal.

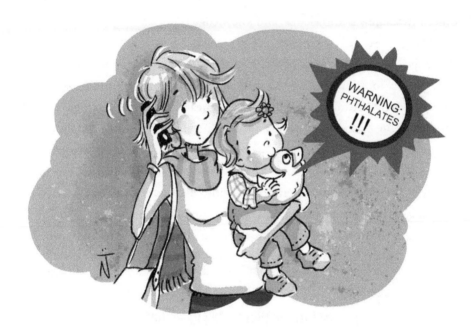

Awareness Is Power

The most common way people give up their
power is by thinking they don't have any.
—Alice Walker

As mothers it's easy for us to recognize when something has an immediate health effect on our children. For example, if we know our child has a peanut allergy and has been exposed to a peanut, we expect immediate reactions like a rash, swelling, or difficulty breathing. Our awareness of the cause and effect of the situation empowers us to protect our children from potential harm.

It's far more difficult to see or understand a connection to a food, household product, or medication when the health effect doesn't take place until days, months, or even years after exposure. Understanding long-term health effects can help us make better choices. Fewer people are smoking these days and more and more people are using sunscreen. Why? Because we now know that over time certain behaviors (smoking and sun exposure) increase our risk for some types of cancer. Awareness is knowledge, and knowledge is power.

Many consumers, including children, are just now beginning to experience the long-term health effects of many modern-day practices and conveniences. Take plastic, for example. We use it in all types of consumer products because it's lightweight, sturdy, convenient, and cheap. However, research recently conducted on plastic has found that certain types of plastics contain a toxic chemical known as bisphenol A (BPA) which may have long-term harmful effects on not only human health, especially our hormones, but the health of our entire ecosystem. When plastic with BPA (plastic coded #3 or #7 for recycling) is heated up (in the microwave or just from hot food sitting on plastic) the BPA can leach out into whatever the plastic item holds, which is often food or drink we consume.

A SOLUTION THAT WASN'T (CHRISTINE)

Back and forth I went to the pediatricians with Kaleigh for an array of problems. Just before her first birthday, the eczema on her face had gotten progressively worse and she'd continued to scratch her face until it bled. They suggested a new prescription cream for the eczema. When I went to pick up the prescription, I instinctively felt uneasy, but I was really hoping this would be the solution. After applying the cream only once, I read the package insert and realized there wasn't any information specifically on use in infants. Although I knew the cream could help her eczema, I was oddly uncomfortable with it and I never used it again. A few years passed before I learned that the cream was pulled from the shelves because it was linked to cancer. It was later put back on the market, but included an FDA box warning about its association with cancer and was no longer recommended for use in children under the age of two.

Recently surfaced, long-term health effects are partly why there are *so many recalls* on household products, food, and medication. Thankfully, awareness of a problem usually leads to safer consumer products. So, if we already *know* that a chemical like BPA is potentially harmful, why are manufacturers still permitted to use it in plastic water bottles, canned goods, and many other consumer products that could potentially end up putting BPA in our children's bodies or our own?

Did You Know?

 Manufacturers voluntarily removed BPA from products such as baby bottles, toddler sippy cups, and infant formula packaging *long before* the FDA's decision to ban BPA from these products in 2012 and 2013. Consumer advocacy groups fought to make sure our infants and toddlers were safer by pressuring stores and manufacturers not to sell baby bottles that used plastic containing BPA. Adding to the pressure was a growing number of chemical safety laws that many states had enacted. This victory is an example of business manufacturers acting responsibly and with integrity, by addressing consumer demands for safer products *before* the FDA mandated it.

Who Holds the Power? Industry and Political Influences

With power comes great responsibility.
—Francois-Marie Arouet aka Voltaire

It's important to remember that many different advocacy groups are out there helping to protect us and that not all businesses or industries are at fault. However, a large part of why we've lost some of our power as consumers is due to industry influence in politics. Some of the largest industries in our country have gotten so big that they appear to have become more powerful than the government agencies set up to monitor them.

For example, no health or safety studies have been required by companies in order for a chemical to be approved for use in the United States. This is due to one of the weakest American environmental laws on the books, known as the Toxic Substances Control Act (TSCA) of 1976. Under TSCA, 62,000 chemicals were "grandfathered in" when the law was enacted and therefore "presumed" to be safe unless the EPA or someone else could *prove* otherwise. Since 1976, the EPA has been successful in banning or restricting only five chemicals. Even as the link between certain chemical exposures and human disease grows, the EPA has had little power to protect us under this law. For example, the EPA was unsuccessful in its attempt to ban asbestos even though it's known to cause cancer. Because of this, eighteen states have passed their *own* chemical safety laws.

Finally, in June of 2016, we made a step in the right direction when President Obama signed a bill to reform the TSCA—The Frank R. Lautenberg Chemical Safety for the 21st Century Act (TSCA Reform), giving the EPA some power to begin to address health and safety concerns on new and existing chemicals on the market. Although the TSCA reform strengthens the EPA's power to protect us, it is far from the solution we deserve. Under the new law, it will take hundreds of years for the EPA to make health and safety assessments for the tens of thousands of untested chemicals already on the market. This clearly demonstrates the political strong arm industry wields. Consumer-driven campaigns that pressure companies to replace harmful chemicals with safer ones may bring about faster change than what we can expect under the new reform. See the Resource Guide (in Part 3 or at www.behindcloseddoorsthebook.com) for more information on TSCA reform.

Europe continues to set the standard for chemical safety, as it operates under the *precautionary principle*. The protection of human health and the environment comes first, and the burden of proof of safety falls on the chemical producers. This means that companies must be able to show that products and the chemicals they contain are safe before they are allowed on store shelves.

Here in the United States, *state laws* will continue to lead the way for some of strongest chemical regulations we have. The states of California and Washington are prime examples.

We need to continue to strengthen the EPA's power and resources to get dangerous chemicals off the market and out of consumer products as quickly as possible. It's too easy to think about our problems in the abstract, but there's nothing vague about the long-term effects of environmental toxins.

WHO PAYS THE PRICE? (JOANNE)

In late 2001, I read a newspaper article about a settlement reached between sixty-nine families in Toms River, New Jersey; two chemical companies; and a water company. According to New Jersey registry data, between 1979 and 1995, ninety children in Toms River were diagnosed with cancer, an abnormally high number. The families blamed the companies for environmental pollution, which they believe resulted in many of the cases of childhood cancers in their community. All three companies agreed to the settlement, but admitted no guilt. The town would later be identified as a childhood cancer cluster during this time period, and contamination from a local chemical plant was identified as the likely source.

The news hit me very hard because I knew some of these kids and their families. While Patrick was going through treatments at CHOP, we'd gotten to know several families from Toms River, and the children we met had both brain tumors and leukemia. After a while, we stopped seeing them, and I got a deeply uneasy feeling; when you stop seeing families at the hospital, far too often you learn that someone has passed away.

Of course all three companies settled these cases but admitted no guilt. How can companies continually get away with toxic pollution, contamination, and cover-ups? The town's drinking water had been contaminated with toxic chemicals, and innocent and unsuspecting families paid the price.

I started thinking about the street I grew up on. During my childhood, many who lived on my street were diagnosed with cancer. At least seven I can easily recall. Many others around town were also diagnosed with cancer and other health issues in numbers that seemed unusually high. Was there some environmental contamination going on in my hometown when I was growing up?

Transparency Problems

> *America will never be destroyed from the outside. If we falter*
> *and lose our freedoms, it will be because we destroyed ourselves.*
> —Abraham Lincoln

An important first step to changing direction is acknowledging that, somewhere along the line, we've abdicated our power to make informed decisions that impact the health of our children. We haven't *willingly* handed this power over to others, but we often haven't been given the necessary information to make educated choices. Many of us have been so caught up in the fast pace of our daily lives that we haven't even noticed what is happening. No clear labeling is required to indicate when food items have been genetically modified or sprayed with toxic pesticides and herbicides. Nor is labeling required when hormones or antibiotics are given to livestock or when their nourishment includes chemical fillers and genetically modified feed.

All of these questionable practices can undermine the integrity of the food system, but are permissible under our current laws or regulations because of industry influence on food policies. It wouldn't be "good for business" if certain information was fully disclosed on food labels, but all of the potential health *effects* of these practices are present in the food we offer our children. Why are more and more young girls going into puberty at a much earlier age? Why have peanut allergies in children tripled? Why has the number of foodborne illnesses skyrocketed from under 7 million cases a year in 1990 to *48 million* cases a year today? *Why* have we accepted many of our current food protocols? Don't we have a right to know all of the practices and ingredients that go into the food we're putting into our children's bodies? Yes, absolutely we do!

Did You Know?

U.S. dairy milk *may* contain genetically-modified hormones unless it's labeled "NO rBGH." Genetically-engineered bovine growth hormone (rBGH) in milk is linked to increased cancer risks—among other health effects—yet some American dairy farmers still inject rBGH into dairy cows to increase milk production. European nations and Canada have already banned rBGH to protect citizens from possible health hazards. Buying organic milk will also guarantee that your milk is 100 percent rBGH free.

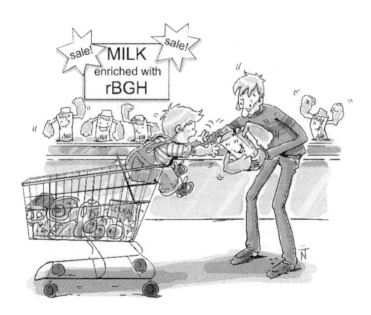

Food isn't the only product lacking transparency for consumers. Trying to avoid a dangerous cancer-causing chemical like formaldehyde is also far more difficult than it should be. Formaldehyde is widely used in a variety of household items, such as pressed wood products, personal care products, and cosmetics. Formadehyde can be listed under *seven* different names on a label (e.g., formalin, methanal, or methylene glycol). This is a tactic often used by manufacturers to avoid unwanted consumer attention. Is this a fair practice? If your child has a formaldehyde allergy or sensitivity, this lack of transparency equals a lack of power to protect them.

The good news is that we have the power to change the way things are. The bottom line is that we shouldn't have to read labels to see if a product is safe for our children. They should be protected from harm by stronger chemical regulations and laws. We can make an immediate difference in the lives of our own children through more educated choices. But we also have an opportunity to stand together and make a difference for *all* children and future generations of children by changing our laws, which is where real and meaningful change takes place.

The next chapter is a snapshot of the changing state of our children's health in this country. For some readers it may be a real eye-opener to learn where we stand as a nation in regard to our children's health and well-being when compared to just a few decades ago. We hope this information will inspire you to want to make changes and to want to work collectively to find solutions to the underlying problems. This chapter will be followed by Part 2, where we take a much deeper and more detailed look at many current industry practices impacting the problem. We will also share the personal experiences of some of the many mothers we met over the last few years. Every voice helps to broaden our discussions and inspire new solutions.

Chapter 3

THE CHANGING STATE OF CHILDREN'S HEALTH

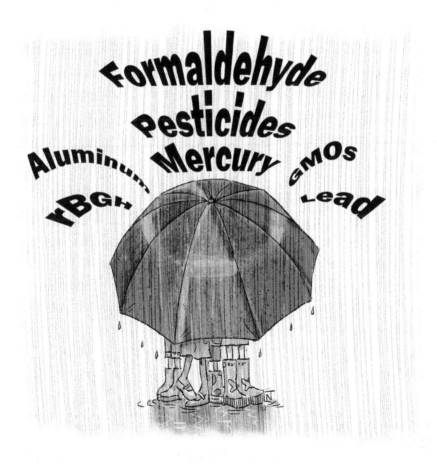

Healthy citizens are the greatest asset any country can have.
—Winston Churchill

WE'RE NUMBER *WHAT*? (JOANNE)

As we began our research, one of our important tasks was to see if there actually had been a rise in children's health conditions over the past few decades. When first setting out to do this, I had no idea how difficult it would be to find current health statistics for children, let alone come up with them from twenty to thirty years ago for comparison.

My background in public health also made me curious about how we compared to other countries in both the health and well-being of children and mothers—so I decided to look into U.S. infant and maternal mortality statistics. When I did, I immediately called Christine and said, "Do you have any idea where the United States ranks among other countries in infant mortality? That's how many infants die during the first year of life."

"I don't know," Christine said. "I'm sure we're right up there, among the top three in the world?"

"Guess again."

"We aren't in the top three?"

"We rank fifty-seventh! That means that fifty-six other countries have lower or better rates of infant mortality than the United States. Our child mortality rate is just as bad in comparison to other nations, and don't even get me started on maternal mortality, which is the worst of all. This is unacceptable! Certainly we can do better than this! What are these other countries doing that we aren't?"

Christine said nothing, before quietly responding, "Maybe the real question is, what are we doing that all these other countries aren't?"

When we compared children's health statistics from today to those from just a few decades ago we found increases in just about every health disorder we explored. Naturally, some proved to be more alarming than others, including the skyrocketing number of children with behavioral health disorders such as autism, ADHD, and bipolar disorder. We also found large increases in the number of children suffering from conditions such as diabetes, obesity, arthritis, and food allergies. The end result is that chronic disease and disability in U.S. children are now at an all-time high. A few decades ago it was rare for a child to have cancer or a life-threatening food allergy; today it is becoming far too common.

We realize that statistics are not everyone's cup of tea. However, the graphs presented in this chapter are vital to understanding the many changes that have occurred in our country and the overall effects of these changes on our children's health. They also serve to support the fundamental premise of our book:

- That many of our children suffer from *chronic* health problems
- That it *wasn't* always like this
- That the problem is *growing*

Below is a summary graphic highlighting some of the most notable increases we found in childhood health disorders over the past few decades. More detailed graphs regarding these statistics and many others follow.

Changes in U.S. Children's Health Over the Past Few Decades

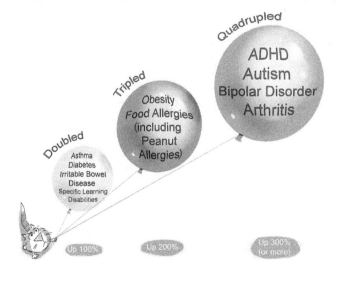

Feel free to browse, at your own pace, the more detailed graphs and related information that follow. Or you can simply skip ahead to the next chapter where we will discuss our findings. Before you begin, we have highlighted a few important points about health statistics and how to interpret our graphs. More information regarding children's health statistics can be found in the Resource Guide in Part 3 or at www.behindcloseddoorsthebook.com.

 A Little Background Information

- Most childhood illnesses or disorders are *not* being tracked on a national level for incidence or prevalence (the number of new or new and existing cases), especially those that only affect a small number of children.

- Often data from a small study published here or there is all that's available for certain children's health conditions, providing a very general estimate of the number of children affected.

- Comparing any health statistic over time poses many different challenges.

- Sometimes even the definition of a childhood condition can change over the period of time health data is compared (*autism* vs. *autism spectrum disorder*). Therefore, an "apples-to-apples" comparison is not always possible.

- Health data takes time (often years) to be collected, analyzed, and published. As a result, a 2014 health statistic may be the most up-to-date statistical data available to use in 2017.

How to Interpret the Graphs

Please know that the graphs and the statistical data derived from the graphs are meant to provide *general estimates* of changes in various U.S. children's health conditions over the past few decades.

Each bar graph will attempt to show the comparison of the number of children diagnosed with a health condition today vs. the number of children diagnosed with the same condition twenty to thirty years ago. Sometimes the study data used in the graphs provide easy and clear comparisons, other times study data provided more challenging comparisons. Therefore, in an effort to provide both transparency and simplicity, we used an apple-to-apple, and apple-to-orange icon system.

If the data being compared over time was essentially the same (from the same study or the same survey) an *apple-to-apple* icon was used. If the data being compared was from different studies or was challenging (because definitions or diagnostic tools changed) then an *apple-to-orange* icon was used. For certain children's health disorders an apple-to-orange comparison was the best we could do because it was the *only* data available within the time period we needed.

Following each graph, you will see bulleted text providing additional information regarding either the studies that support the graph or the particular children's health condition displayed. In-graph citations are provided. Full references can be found in Part 3 of this book. And for the most up-to-date data, see www.behindcloseddoorsthebook.com.

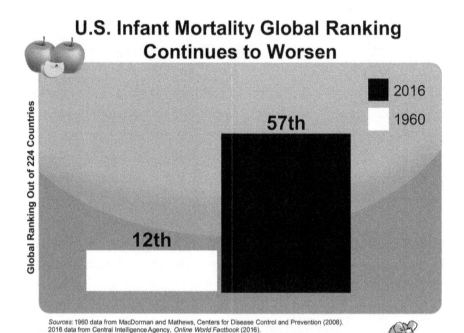

U.S. Infant Mortality Global Ranking Continues to Worsen

Global Ranking Out of 224 Countries

2016 · **1960**

57th

12th

Sources: 1960 data from MacDorman and Mathews, Centers for Disease Control and Prevention (2008).
2016 data from Central Intelligence Agency, *Online World Factbook* (2016).

"Infant mortality is one of the most important indicators of the health of a nation, as it is associated with a variety of factors such as maternal health, quality and access to medical care, socioeconomic conditions, and public health practices."
- *U.S. Centers for Disease Control & Prevention*

▷ Infant mortality is defined as the number of deaths in infants under the age of one year. The 2016 estimate for U.S. infant mortality rate was 5.8 per 1,000 live births.

▷ Today, 56 countries boast lower infant mortality rates than the United States. Although our infant mortality rates have improved drastically since 1960 - we are not keeping up with the progress of other countries.

▷ According to the Centers for Disease Control and Prevention (CDC), most infant deaths are attributed to birth defects, preterm delivery, maternal complications of pregnancy, sudden infant death syndrome (SIDS), and injuries (e.g., suffocation).

▷ According to 2015 CDC data, African Americans have double the rate of infant deaths as non-Hispanic Whites. Lack of access to healthcare is one contributing factor.

▷ Babies born prematurely have played a key role in infant mortality. According to a 2013 special report in *Stanford Medicine*, although fertility treatments and teenage pregnancies both raise the risk of preterm births, neither explains the diversity in infant mortality rates, as states with high infant mortality have no higher rates of either fertility or teen pregnancies.

▷ A 2000 study by the National Research Council found that 50% of all pregnancies in the United States were resulting in prenatal or postnatal mortality; significant birth defects; developmental, neurological, or immune conditions; or otherwise chronically unhealthy babies.

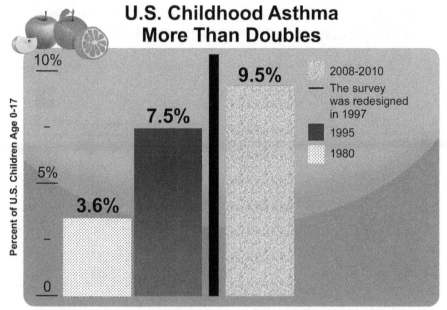

U.S. Childhood Asthma More Than Doubles

Sources: 1980-1995 data from Akinbami, Centers for Disease Control and Prevention (2006). 2008-2010 data from Centers for Disease Control and Prevention, *NCHS Data Brief* (2012).
Notes: The National Health Interview Survey was used by sources to track asthma prevalence from 1980-2010. The survey questions for asthma changed in 1997; therefore data prior to 1997 cannot be directly compared to data after 1997.

▷ Asthma is the most common chronic illness in U.S. children and causes 14 million missed school days each year. Asthma places a huge hardship on affected children and their families.

▷ It is known that pollutants in the air can trigger asthma. However, various other sources of environmental toxins found in food, water, and household products can also be triggers.

▷ Toxins not only cause inflammation in the body but they also breakdown our immune system and its ability to detoxify itself. The immune system creates all allergies and allergies create most asthma in children.

▷ Examples of other asthma triggers include: allergens, infections, exercise, changes in the weather, and exposure to airway irritants.

▷ Decreasing your child's exposure to triggers will help decrease symptoms as well as the need for asthma medications. Some of the necessary treatments for asthma such as anti-inflammatories and bronchodilators can pose other future health problems when taken for an extended period of time.

Study Reflects Nearly 300% Increase in Food Allergy Outpatient Visits Among U.S. Children

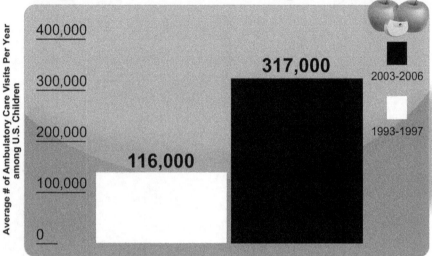

Source: Data from Branum and Lukacs, *Pediatrics* (2009).

Note: The same study also reflects an over 350% increase in the number of food allergy related hospitalizations for U.S. children between 1998-2000 and 2004-2006.

⇨ A food allergy is a potentially serious immune response to eating specific foods or food additives.

⇨ Children with a food allergy are 2 to 4 times more likely to have other related conditions such as asthma and other allergies, compared with children without food allergies.

⇨ Parents should become familiar with the early signs of allergic reactions such as eczema, hives, wheezing, and repeated diarrhea and/or vomiting in reaction to formulas or foods.

⇨ A child may be allergic to a food even if the child has eaten it many times before without a problem because it may take days, weeks, or longer to build up enough immune response to cause noticeable symptoms.

⇨ Many of our foods have become highly refined over the years. Foods are also filled with food additives and genetic modifications. All have been theorized as possible culprits to the large rise in food allergies.

⇨ The rise in food allergies starting in the mid-1990s coincides with the adoption of genetically modified food in the U.S.

⇨ Peanut is the most prevalent food allergen in children, followed by milk, and then shellfish.

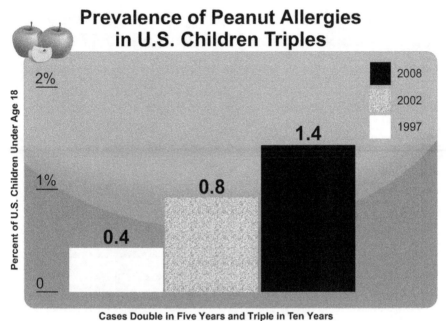

Prevalence of Peanut Allergies in U.S. Children Triples

Percent of U.S. Children Under Age 18

2008
2002
1997

2%

1%

0

0.4
0.8
1.4

Cases Double in Five Years and Triple in Ten Years

Source: Data from Sicherer et al., Journal of Allergy and Clinical Immunology (2010).

⇨ A peanut allergy occurs when your immune system mistakenly identifies peanut proteins as something harmful.

⇨ A peanut allergy, unlike other food allergies, is seldom outgrown.

⇨ Since January 2006, foods covered by the FDA labeling laws that contain peanuts must be labeled to declare that it "contains peanut." However, there are many foods and products not covered by FDA allergen labeling laws, so it is still important to know how to read a label for peanut ingredients. For instance, highly processed peanut oil is exempt from allergen labeling laws.

⇨ There are several theories concerning the rise of peanut allergies in children, including the way peanuts are processed and the fact that children are not being exposed to peanuts at a young enough age. The American Academy of Pediatrics used to instruct parents to avoid peanut use until their children reached age 3, but that has since been rescinded.

⇨ Another theory for the general rise in both peanut and food allergies is the "hygiene theory." This theory suggests we have become cleaner and less healthy due to the use of antibacterial products in the home as well as the increased use of vaccinations and antibiotics in medicine. This may throw the immune system off balance and impair the development of a healthy (diverse) bacterial microbiome in the gut. This makes the immune system more reactive and less able to differentiate real vs. harmless threats (like food).

Incidence of Inflammatory Bowel Disease Doubles among Children age 0-17

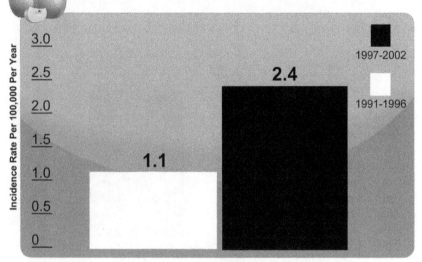

Studied Cohorts of Children Registered in the IBD Center at Texas Children's Hospital
Source: Data from Malaty, Journal of Pediatric Gastroenterology and Nutrition (2010).

▷ Inflammatory bowel disease (IBD) refers to a group of chronic diseases, of which Crohn's disease and ulcerative colitis are the 2 main types.

▷ Research suggests that the cause of IBD is a combination of 3 main factors: genetics, the immune system, and the environment.

▷ One of the most important issues that needs to be addressed specifically in children with IBD is a lack of growth.

▷ The study used in our graph revealed that white children had a higher risk for IBD compared with Hispanic and African American children studied.

▷ The study reflected the highest increase in incidence of IBD was among the 10-12 year-old age group.

▷ A 2013 study, published in the *Journal of Investigative Medicine,* found a 65% increase in IBD hospitalizations from 2000 to 2009.

▷ Although the reasons behind the rise of childhood IBD remain unclear, genetic makeup does not change drastically in populations over short periods of time, therefore it is likely that changing environmental factors are triggering new cases in genetically predisposed children.

U.S. Childhood Obesity Prevalence Triples

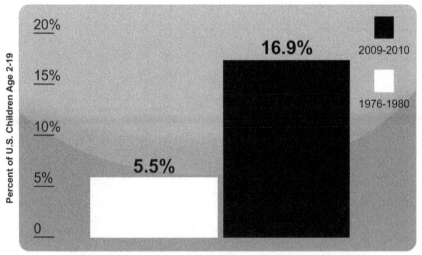

Percent of U.S. Children Age 2-19

20%

15%

10%

5%

0

16.9% 2009-2010

1976-1980

5.5%

12.5 Million U.S. Children and Adolescents Age 2-19 Years Are Obese

Sources: 1976-1980 data from Ogden and Carroll, Centers for Disease Control and Prevention (2010). 2009-2010 data from Centers for Disease Control and Prevention, *NCHS Fact Sheet* (2012).
Note: Obesity defined as body mass index (BMI) greater than or equal to sex- and age-specific 95th percentile from the 2000 CDC Growth Charts.

▷ By 2008, 1 out of every 3 children or adolescents in the United States was considered to be overweight or obese.

▷ Excess weight is the single greatest risk factor for Type 2 diabetes in children.

▷ One of the best ways to combat obesity is increasing opportunities for children to engage in physical activity.

▷ According to the CDC, childhood obesity has both immediate and long-term health impacts including an increased risk of developing cardiovascular disease, bone and joint problems, sleep apnea, and social and psychological problems such as stigmatization and poor self-esteem.

▷ Endocrine disruptor is a term used to describe the impact of various chemicals in food, consumer products, and the environment that either mimic or block hormones and disrupt the body's normal functions. Many have also been identified as "obesogens"; specific chemicals that not only disrupt the endocrine system but also promote weight gain and obesity.

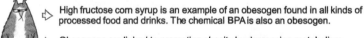

▷ High fructose corn syrup is an example of an obesogen found in all kinds of processed food and drinks. The chemical BPA is also an obesogen.

▷ Obesogens are linked to promoting obesity by decreasing metabolism, increasing fat cells, and altering the brain's ability to manage feelings of hunger.

Mental Health Disorders

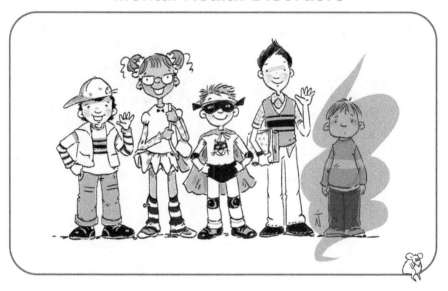

1 out of every 5 children in the United States has a mental health disorder.

In the late 1990s we began to see increases in mental health medications prescribed to children, giving us our first clue that more children were being diagnosed with mental health disorders. Between 1995 and 1998 the use of antidepressants, mood stabilizers, and antipsychotics in children skyrocketed. For example, the use of antidepressants in children under age 6 had increased by 580%.

Mental Health
now accounts for the most dollars spent
on children's health in the United States

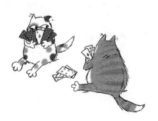

Depression

Although we could not locate a specific study that adequately compared depression incidence in United States children over the past few decades to present a graph, we can share the following information about depression among U.S. children and young adults.

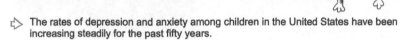

▷ The rates of depression and anxiety among children in the United States have been increasing steadily for the past fifty years.

▷ A Harvard study estimated that the rate of depression among children was increasing by 23% a year.

▷ A study examining trends in prescription drugs revealed that preschoolers (age 0-5) are the fastest growing market for antidepressant medication.

▷ According to a 2010 study, there are now 5 to 8 times as many high school and college students in the United States meeting the criteria for diagnosis of major depression and/or an anxiety disorder compared to 50 years ago.

▷ A 2009 U.S. high school student survey showed that 13.8% of students in grades 9-12 seriously considered suicide in the previous 12 months and 6.3% of students reported making at least one suicide attempt in the previous 12 months.

▷ The FDA has placed a "black box" warning label — the most serious type of warning — on all antidepressant medications. The warning says there is an increased risk of suicidal thinking or attempts in youth taking antidepressants. Many antidepressants cause additional serious side effects.

▷ The FDA warns that some ADHD medications may lead to depression many years after the medication has been administered.

▷ According to the American Academy of Child and Adolescent Psychiatry, both genetics and the environment play a role in depression. Depression in children can be triggered by things such as a medical illness, a stressful situation, or the loss of an important person. Sometimes it is difficult to identify a triggering event.

▷ Some of the chemicals children are exposed to are considered to be neuro-toxins (toxic to the brain). Therefore, research into possible causes of children's mental health disorders may need to begin to include toxicology, environmental sciences, and occupational medicine. These are science disciplines that all study toxicological causes of disease including mental health disease.

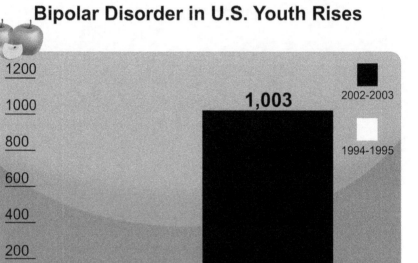

Bipolar Disorder in U.S. Youth Rises

Office Visits Per 100,000 U.S. Children

1200

1000

800

600

400

200

0

1,003

2002-2003

1994-1995

25

Visits That Diagnosed the Disorder Increased 40-Fold

Source: Data from Moreno et al., *Archives of General Psychiatry* (2007).

▷ Children with bipolar disorder experience unusually intense shifts in mood characterized by a complex and continuous cycling of mania (euphoria) and depression.

▷ The extreme highs and lows of mood are accompanied by extreme changes in energy, activity, sleep, and behavior.

▷ Studies suggest that the majority of bipolar disorder cases in children are chronic.

▷ Children diagnosed with bipolar disorder often suffer from an additional, coexisting mental health condition such as ADHD, depression, or psychosis.

▷ Medicating children for bipolar disorder can present many challenges and children need to be monitored closely for any changes in behavior when starting or stopping medication.

▷ According to a CDC report, in 2010 mood disorders were among the most common principal diagnosis for all hospital stays among children in the United States, with the rate of hospital stays among children for mood disorders increasing 80% during 1997-2010.

▷ Suicide, which can result from the interaction of mental health disorders and other factors, was the second leading cause of death among children age 12-17 in 2010.

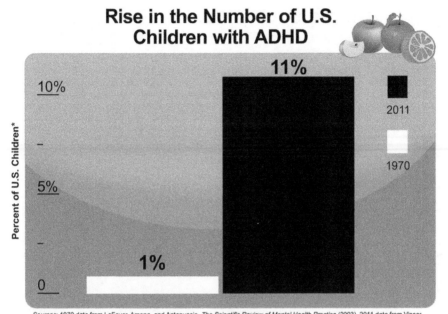

Rise in the Number of U.S. Children with ADHD

11%

10%

Percent of U.S. Children*

5%

1%

0

2011

1970

Sources: 1970 data from LeFever, Arcona, and Antonuccio, *The Scientific Review of Mental Health Practice* (2003). 2011 data from Visser et al., *Journal of the American Academy of Child & Adolescent Psychiatry* (2014).
Notes: The diagnostic criteria for ADHD changed from 1970 to 2007-2009. In 1970 there was no ADHD diagnosis and the studies 1% estimate derives from prescription Ritalin™ use at the time. *1970 study prevalence percentage was based on number of U.S. schoolchildren in that year. 2011 prevalence data was based on the National Survey of Children's Health (NSCH) for children aged 4-17 years. The NSCH was not available in 1970 for direct comparision.

- ADHD symptoms may include difficulty staying focused and paying attention, restlessness, difficulty controlling behavior, hyperactivity (overactivity), and disorganization.

- A 2015 study conducted by the CDC on ADHD treatment in children revealed that 25% of U.S. toddlers taking ADHD medication were doing so without having tried behavioral interventions first. Behavioral interventions are proven to be safe while the long-term effects of psychotropic medications on the developing mind and body of young children are unknown.

- Studies show that ADHD may result from exposure to environmental contaminants such as lead, methyl mercury, brominated flame retardants, and PCBs as either a fetus or as a young child.

- A recent study of U.S. children found that children exposed to organophosphate chemicals from pesticides on commercially grown fruits and vegetables were more likely to have ADHD than children with less exposure. Organophosphate pesticides (OP) are designed to kill pests by having a toxic effect on the nervous system. Even at low levels, OP exposure may be harmful to the brain development of fetuses and young children.

- Food preservatives BHA (butylated hydroxyanisole), BHT (butylated hydroxytoluene), and TBHQ (tertiary butylhydroquinone) have been found to trigger behavioral and health problems.

- There are over 15 published studies that link artificial food dyes to ADHD. Europe requires labels on food containing certain suspected food dyes, but not in the U.S.

A Little Background on Diabetes

The earliest childhood diabetes estimates in the United States are from the 1960s-1990s and originated from a few select registries at state and local levels in areas such as Philadelphia and Wisconsin. These small geographic snapshots provided us with our first glimpse into the estimated number of U.S. children with a diagnosis of Type I diabetes.

In the year 2000, in response to the growing public concern about a rise in U.S. children with diabetes (both Type 1 and Type 2), the Centers for Disease Control and Prevention (CDC) and the National Institute of Health (NIH) launched the SEARCH for Diabetes Study, which is a national multicenter study aimed at understanding more about diabetes among children and young adults in the United States.

Type 1 and Type 2 Diabetes: What's the difference?

Type I diabetes was formerly known as *juvenile-onset diabetes*. In Type 1 diabetes, a child's own body has destroyed its ability to produce insulin, resulting in a permanent deficiency of insulin needed to regulate blood sugar. There is no cure for Type 1 diabetes.

Type 2 diabetes was formerly known as *adult-onset diabetes* but is now commonly affecting children. In Type 2 diabetes, a child's body does not use the insulin it makes effectively (insulin resistance), disrupting the regulation of blood sugar. One of the biggest risk factors for Type 2 diabetes in children is being overweight. Type 2 diabetes can often be controlled with a healthy diet and exercise and does not usually require daily insulin.

Our diabetes graph uses incidence data from the early registry in Wisconsin because it provides reliable data to compare over the last few decades. It was also consistent with increases in Type 1 diabetes found in the Philadelphia registry over the past 20 years. We did not include Type 2 diabetes graphs because the increases in this disorder are closely related to the large increases in childhood obesity already presented.

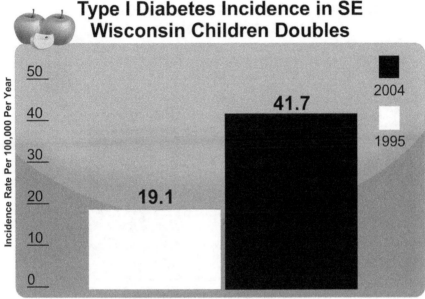

Type I Diabetes Incidence in SE Wisconsin Children Doubles

Incidence Rate Per 100,000 Per Year

50

40 — **41.7**

30

20 — **19.1**

10

0

■ 2004

□ 1995

Studied Children Age 0-19 from the Children's Hospital of Wisconsin Diabetes Center

Source: Data from Evertsen, Alemzadeh, Wang, *PLoS ONE* (2009).

⇨ Type 1 diabetes is an autoimmune disorder that will typically strike children and young adults and those affected will require the use of daily insulin injections or an insulin pump to survive.

⇨ The exact cause of Type 1 diabetes is still unclear. However, it is believed that Type 1 diabetes results from injuries due to an infection or toxins in children whose immune system is predisposed to developing diabetes.

⇨ According to the CDC, autoimmune, genetic, and environmental factors are involved in children developing Type 1 diabetes.

⇨ A diagnosis of Type 1 diabetes (juvenile diabetes) will decrease a child's life expectancy by 15 years.

⇨ Children with diabetes are at great risk of developing serious long-term health complications such as heart disease, kidney disease, blindness, and stroke.

⇨ The most rapid increases in Type 1 diabetes is being seen in children age 0-4, putting our youngest children at the highest risk for death due to an often delayed diagnosis. Are the increasing number of environmental toxins our children are exposed to taxing the developing immune system and contributing to this rise?

Juvenile Arthritis in U.S. Children Increases 9-Fold

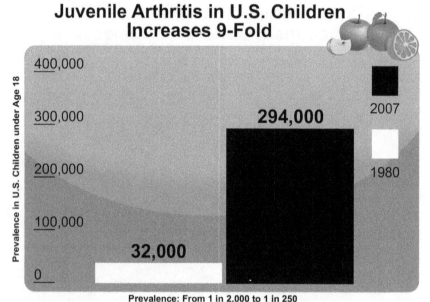

Prevalence in U.S. Children under Age 18

400,000

300,000 — **294,000** — 2007

200,000 — 1980

100,000

32,000

0

Prevalence: From 1 in 2,000 to 1 in 250

Sources: 1980 data from Gewanter, Roghmann, and Baum, *Arthritis & Rheumatism* (1983). 2007 data from Centers for Disease Control and Prevention (2010).
Notes: 2007 data was the first year the CDC provided national estimates and included juvenile arthritis and other childhood arthritis related diagnoses. Diagnosis methods and definitions may have varied from 1980 and 2007 making comparisons difficult.

⟁ Juvenile Arthritis (JA) is one of the most common chronic childhood diseases that often go undetected or misdiagnosed.

⟁ JA can impede a child's ability to partake in daily living activities such as dressing, walking, or playing sports.

⟁ JA is an autoimmune disorder, which means that the body's own immune system starts to attack and destroy cells and tissues (particularly in the joints) for no apparent reason. It is believed that the immune system can be provoked by changes in the genes or the environment.

⟁ There has been no causal relationship established between food and arthritis proven by large scientific studies. However, a 1990 study published in the *Journal of Rheumatology* concluded that a small number of rheumatic disease patients have "immunologic sensitivity" to food.

⟁ Manufacturer's vaccination product inserts report a possible association between arthritis and the hepatitis 8, rubella, MMR, varicella, and HPV vaccinations.

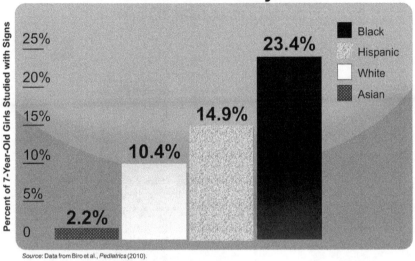

2010 Study Reveals Signs of Early Puberty in 7-Year-Old Girls by Race

Source: Data from Biro et al., *Pediatrics* (2010).

⇨ A growing number of U.S. girls are developing breast buds and entering into puberty at younger ages compared to 10 to 30 years ago.

⇨ Children with precocious (early) puberty are often under social and psychological stress due to physical and hormonal changes their bodies are undergoing that their mind may be too young to understand.

⇨ Early menstruation in girls is linked to an increased risk for breast cancer and short stature.

⇨ Early puberty may be linked to the increase in childhood obesity, chemicals in processed food, and environmental chemicals that act as endocrine disruptors, such as BPA (a synthetic estrogen that can disrupt the hormone system, often found in plastics and used in the lining of metal canned goods including some infant formulas).

⇨ A 2012 study showed that boys in the United States are also experiencing the onset of early puberty at a younger age. The study revealed that black boys (9.1 years old) were more likely to start puberty earlier than Hispanic (10.0 years old) or white boys (10.1 years old).

Increases in Number of Children Served in U.S. Public School Special Education under IDEA

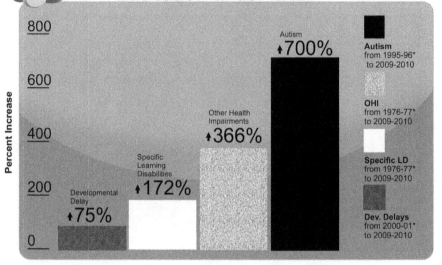

Sources: 1976-2001 data from Aud et al., *U.S. Department of Education* (2010). 2009-2010 data from Aud et al., *U.S. Department of Education* (2012).
Note: The Individuals with Disabilities Education Act (IDEA), enacted in 1975, mandates that children and youth ages 3-21 with disabilities be provided a free and appropriate public school education. Other health impairment means having a disability caused by disease, condition, disorder, or injury that substantially affects strength, vitality, or alertness (i.e., cancer or heart condition).
* Denotes first year data was available

▷ Data from the U.S. Department of Special Education (used in our graph) is usually conservative when compared to the actual number of children in the United States with these disabilities.

▷ A learning disability (LD) is much more than a "difference" or "difficulty" with learning. It is a neurological disorder that affects the brain's ability to receive, process, store, and respond to information.

▷ LDs affect many areas of a child's life - not just school.

▷ Children with LDs are twice as likely to drop out of school and twice as likely to be unemployed in the future vs. a child without an LD.

▷ LDs may be associated with exposure to environmental toxins. Studies estimate that 50% of all children with LDs have higher levels of heavy metals in their bodies including lead and cadmium.

▷ The EPA estimates that more than 300,000 newborns each year in the United States may have increased risk of LDs due to their mother's exposure to methylmercury from fish consumption during pregnancy.

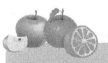

U.S. Autism Prevalence Estimates Continue to Climb

Year	# of Children Affected	Source
Prior to 1980	1 to 4 in every 10,000	NAA and CDC
1995-96	1 in every 1,000	U.S. Dept of Education
1997-99	1 in every 526	CDC/NHIS
2000	1 in every 150	CDC/ADDM Network
2004	1 in every 125	CDC/ADDM Network
2008	1 in every 88	CDC/ADDM Network
2011-12*	1 in every 50	CDC/NSCH

Sources: 1980 and earlier data from *National Autism Association* (2013) and Rice, *CDC Morbidity and Mortality Weekly Report* (2013). 1995-1996 data from Aud et al., *U.S. Department of Education* (2010). 1997-1999 data from Boyle et al., *Pediatrics* (2011). 2000-2008 data from *Centers for Disease Control and Prevention* (2012). The Autism and Developmental Disabilities Monitoring Network. 2011-2012 data from Blumberg et al., *National Health Statistics Report* (2013). *Most up to date statistic at the time of publication. National Survey of Children's Health. *Note*: It is very problematic to compare autism rates over the last three decades, as the diagnostic criteria as well as definitions for autism and autism spectrum disorder (ASD) have changed. Methods of data collection may also have varied.

▷ Approximately 1 in every 50 U.S. children are now being diagnosed with autism or a related disorder.

▷ Autism spectrum disorder (ASD) is a group of developmental disorders that can appear in the first 3 years of life. ASD affects the brain's normal development of social and communication skills.

▷ The cause of autism is unknown. However, according to the National Institute of Health (NIH), there is likely a combination of factors that lead to ASD including both environmental factors and genetic factors.

▷ Early intervention is key, it is important that parents act quickly whenever there is a concern about a child's development. Remember that you do not need a diagnosis to access services for your child.

▷ Many autism parents have found great success with the use of nontraditional medical interventions such as environmental medicine, dietary interventions (e.g., gluten-free and casein-free), and the use of chiropractic care. It is important to find a reputable practitioner when choosing alternative therapies.

▷ Research in the area of autism, including proposed theories behind causes and treatments, is ever evolving. A newer theory acknowledges that although genetics may play a role — the underlying condition may be more of an acquired metabolic (biochemical) syndrome, in which the immune system and the microbiome (primarily gut bacteria) likely play a role.

U.S. Childhood Cancer
Incidence Continues to Rise

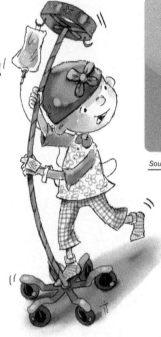

1 in 285 U.S. Children Will Be Diagnosed with Cancer Before the Age of 20

Source: Data from American Cancer Society (2014)

⊳ Between 1975 and 2010 the overall incidence rate of cancer in U.S. children ages 0-14 rose from 11.5 to 16.4 (per 100,000 children).

⊳ Cancer is the #1 cause of death from disease in U.S. children.

⊳ Leukemias and brain tumors are the most common types of childhood cancers. Together they account for almost 50% of all childhood cancers in the United States.

⊳ Exposure to radiation is the major risk factor for childhood cancer. Studies also support a connection between environmental toxins and childhood cancers.

⊳ Today, the survival rate (being alive 5 years after a diagnosis) for childhood cancer surpasses 80%. Survivorship in children is very different than survivorship in adults.

⊳ Children survivors are often left with chronic health conditions as a result of either the cancer itself or the very treatments that saved their lives.

⊳ Late effects from treatment can include heart damage, second cancers, lung damage, infertility, cognitive impairment, growth deficits, hearing loss, and more. They often occur because the cancer and its treatment (which is often highly toxic) occur at a critical time period when a child's body and brain are still growing and developing.

⊳ Finding less toxic treatments for childhood cancer must become a top research priority!

The President's Cancer Panel
The Rise in Childhood Cancer Rates
in the United States

In May of 2010, the President's Cancer Panel provided its annual report and recommendations to the President of the United States. The President's Cancer Panel is a federal advisory committee appointed by the President, charged with monitoring the development and execution of the activities of the National Cancer Program. The President's *Cancer Panel Annual Report* (2010) acknowledged the continual rise in childhood cancer rates and stressed that the proliferation of chemicals in water, foods, air and household products is widely suspected as a factor. Here is what they had to say:

> "It is vitally important to recognize that children are far more susceptible to damage from environmental carcinogens and endocrine-disrupting compounds than adults. To the extent possible, parents and childcare providers should choose foods, house and garden products, play spaces, toys, medicines, and medical tests that will minimize children's exposure to toxics. Ideally, both mothers and fathers should avoid exposures to endocrine-disrupting chemicals and known or suspected carcinogens prior to a child's conception and throughout pregnancy and early life, when risk of damage is greatest."

The panel made recommendations for simple steps we can take to reduce the risk of cancer in our children. These recommendations can be found in the **Resource Guide** in Part 3 of this book.

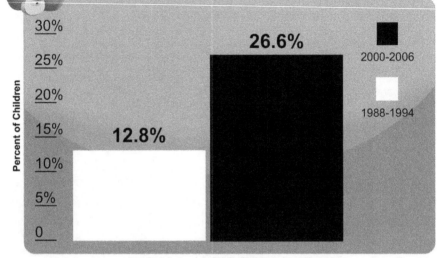

Prevalence of Chronic Health Conditions among U.S. Children age 2-8 Doubles

Percent of Children

30%
25%
20%
15%
10%
5%
0

26.6%

2000-2006

1988-1994

12.8%

Studied Cohorts of U.S. Children for 6 Years

Source: Data from Van Cleave, Gortmaker, and Perrin, *Journal of the American Medical Association* (2010).

⇨ 1 in every 4 children studied in the 2000-2006 cohort had a chronic illness at the end of the study and more than 50% experienced a chronic illness at some point during the study.

⇨ Even more alarming were results of a 2007 National Survey of Children's Health estimating that 43% of U.S. children (32 million) are living with a chronic illness. The percentage rose to 54% of U.S. children when overweight, obesity and being at risk for a developmental delay were included among the chronic health conditions.

⇨ To additionally support the data presented in our graph, the largest U.S. pharmacy benefit manager also reported that more than 25% of U.S. children were taking regular medication based on 2009 data.

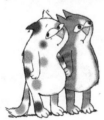

Chapter 4

TRYING TO MAKE SENSE OF IT ALL

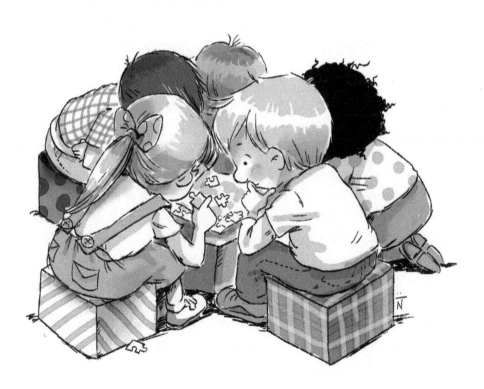

*Children are the world's most valuable resource
and its best hope for our future.*
—John Fitzgerald Kennedy

While compiling these health statistics, we were just as shocked as you may now feel. Who knew the United States had one of the highest rates of infant mortality in the industrialized world? Who knew how chronically ill our nation's children have become? Over the past few decades, we appear to have shifted from a country whose children more commonly suffered from short-term acute illnesses (such as strep throat) to a country whose children are increasingly suffering from long-term chronic illnesses (such as diabetes, asthma, or autism). This shift is a grim issue that needs our attention. Many of us know firsthand that these illnesses have serious medical, social, and financial implications that can affect the entire family. America is only beginning to understand the enormous price tag and burden associated with a chronic disease remaining with a child over a lifetime. For example, many parents of autistic children are only now realizing the challenges they face as eligibility for school special education services ends after age twenty-one. How will these young adults spend their days? Who will care for them? How will those who are able to work get to and from a place of employment if they cannot drive?

Our current health statistics shouldn't be accepted as normal because *it wasn't always like this!* Were school nurses always this overwhelmed? Did school cafeterias always have a separate table for students with food allergies? Did we get our first bras at seven and first periods at nine? Were our childhood friends taking antidepressants? Was childhood obesity an epidemic in neighborhoods where we grew up? Were there always this many kids with autism? Something is wrong when 25 percent of the *children* in our country require daily medications for a chronic illness and when healthcare spending for children is growing at a faster rate than for adults.

A BIG DIFFERENCE (TONI, FIFTH-GRADE TEACHER)

I don't need statistics to tell me we have children's health issues! I laugh when I hear people try to reduce the problem to merely more kids being tested and diagnosed with problems. There is a big difference in the children that fill my classroom today vs. those that filled my classroom twenty years ago. Some days I feel more like a school nurse than a school teacher!

We can't help but wonder if we are doing all we can to research the *cause* of an illness and work towards prevention, instead of focusing so much time and money toward treating the symptoms and simply controlling an illness. Yes, we absolutely want to treat and control chronic health problems, but in the long term we would much rather cure them and better understand how to prevent them in the future. The most important question we need to ask ourselves is, what is the root cause of this shift from acute to chronic illness in our children? When we identify and address the answer to this question, we will begin to see better health for our kids.

It All Adds Up

Our children are exposed to a variety of toxins from various sources on a daily basis. These toxins can break down a body's immune system and, as a result, compromise our children's health, putting them at increased risk for developing illness or disease—especially those that are "autoimmune" in nature. Although it may be unrealistic to think we can provide a completely toxin-free environment for our children, we can reduce their exposure if we are aware of what the harmful substances are and where they can be found. We also need to understand how these exposures may be adding up.

Did You Know?

 Autoimmune disorders occur when the immune system, which is normally involved in defending the body against disease, mistakenly recognizes healthy cells as something foreign. As a result, the body begins to attack and destroy healthy cells and tissue.

As mothers, we're always trying to do what's best for our children. It is a full-time job, and often there doesn't seem to be enough hours in a day. When we do find time to look into something of concern, we can experience *information overload*. Just trying to sort through everything available on the Internet can be confusing and overwhelming, especially when it's conflicting or seems illogical.

For example, the World Health Organization (WHO), the Environmental Protection Agency (EPA), the Food and Drug Administration (FDA), and the Agency for Toxic Substances and Disease Registry (ATSDR) all set different limits on what is a *permissible* or *minimal risk* amount of mercury to have in our food, medicine, and environment. But at least they all agree that mercury is an extremely dangerous chemical element that's highly toxic in small amounts, especially to the brains of a developing fetus, infant, or child.

Yet some of these same government agency websites inform us that a small amount of "necessary" mercury is contained in some consumer products. For example, a small amount of mercury is contained in every new CFL lightbulb (hey, no worries unless it breaks). A small amount of mercury (thimerosal) is *still used* in certain childhood vaccinations (didn't they say it was most toxic to the brain of an infant?). And a small amount of mercury (50 percent mercury content by weight) is used in silver "amalgam" dental fillings that provide a good low-cost option for consumers (safety is only for those who can afford it?).

Recommendations are also made for a "safe" level of the mercury-laden fish we can consume. Naturally, these recommendations are made for our protection, but with all the different forms of mercury and other toxic substances our children are knowingly subjected to, the common sense questions many mothers want to ask are:

- "Who's paying attention to the sum of all the toxins the average American child is exposed to and determining if the *sum* of these exposures is safe?"
- "Are these 'safe' levels based on a child's body weight or an adult's?"
- "What are the long-term health effects of all these combined exposures?"

ATHLETES OF THE NEW MILLENNIUM (JOANNE)

I coached high school and college field hockey on and off for close to twenty years. Working with teenagers and young adults has been one of the most rewarding and joyful experiences of my life. For my first ten years coaching I only had one or two players with any medical concerns. The next ten years were a whole different story. By the 1999–2000 school year, I had a huge plastic bag on the sidelines with me every day that was filled with asthma inhalers, EpiPens, insulin, and other blood sugar–related products—each carefully labeled with one of my player's names. Now sprinkle in a few players with attention-deficit disorder and a few players who had undergone multiple knee surgeries now sporting bulky orthopedic braces. These were the athletes on my team. Not just on my team, this was the athlete of the new millennium. Compromised, yet resilient!

The President's Cancer Panel Agrees

While we were researching for this book, the 2010 President's Cancer Panel report and recommendations to President Obama were released. The report not only supported our motherly intuition but raised it to another level. Below is an excerpt from the report:

Perhaps most importantly, the impact of various exposures, whether individual, simultaneous, sequential, or cumulative over a lifetime, may not be simply additive. Instead, combinations of exposures may have synergistic effects that intensify or otherwise alter their impact compared with the effect of each contaminant alone. In addition, we now recognize that critical periods of time exist across the life span (e.g., prenatal and early life, puberty) when individuals are particularly susceptible to damage from environmental contaminants. Moreover, a person's genetic make-up can significantly affect his or her susceptibility to the harmful effects of an environmental agent, and it also is becoming clear that some exposures can have effects across multiple generations.

The many experts in academia who collaborated with the President's Cancer Panel (PCP) know that exposure to toxic chemicals poses a serious health risk to children and that this needs to be brought to the public's attention. Here is an excerpt from the PCP's letter to President Obama that accompanied the report:

> The Panel was particularly concerned to find that the true burden of environmentally induced cancer has been grossly underestimated. With nearly 80,000 chemicals on the market in the United States, many of which are used by millions of Americans in their daily lives and are un- or understudied and largely unregulated, exposure to potential environmental carcinogens is widespread. . . .
>
> Most also are unaware that children are far more vulnerable to environmental toxins and radiation than adults. Efforts to inform the public of such harmful exposures and how to prevent them must be increased. All levels of government, from federal to local, must work to protect every American from needless disease through rigorous regulation of environmental pollutants.

If the experts and now the president of the United States are aware of so many risks to children from various environmental factors, why do they continue? Other countries have banned health-threatening chemicals commonly found in U.S. food, household goods, and health and beauty products. To protect their citizens these nations have removed potentially harmful products and protocols, while in the United States the very same products and protocols are still considered "safe" under various laws, regulations, or guidelines.

It's time to go behind the closed doors of industry and politics to see how our everyday practices and laws may be contributing to some of the health issues in our children. In Part 2, we will explore the possible causes of these problems, examine our options, and together work towards solutions.

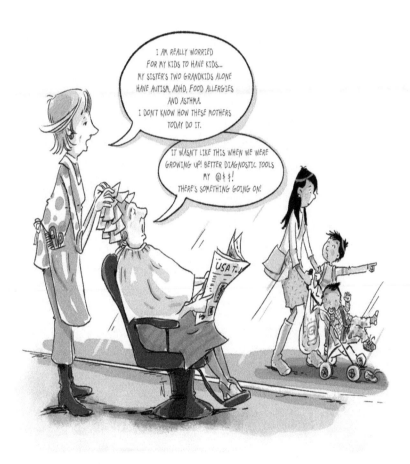

GOING BEHIND CLOSED DOORS

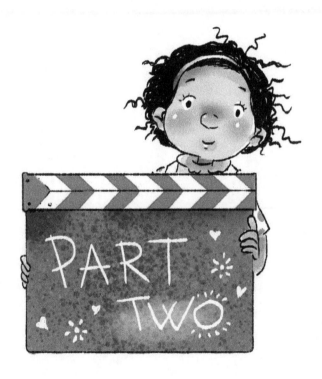

Chapter 5

THE FOOD INDUSTRY

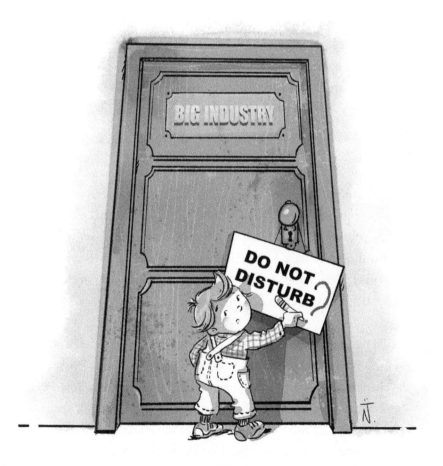

Don't eat anything your great-grandmother wouldn't recognize as food.
—Michael Pollan

GOODBYE SUPERMARKET SHELF (CHRISTINE)

"Kaleigh can have nothing to eat from a can or a box."

This was the advice from our allergy doctor after he read me the list of her food allergies: wheat, dairy, eggs, bananas, seafood, and peanuts.

He then warned, "Her seafood and peanut allergy can be life-threatening and she should always carry an EpiPen."

"How did this happen?" I asked, barraging him with questions. "What's causing these food allergies? How can we fix this?"

While he didn't have the answers, his advice and direction regarding avoidance of all processed food was lifesaving for Kaleigh. In addition to her food allergies, Kaleigh had also experienced sensitivities to many different chemical additives. His words led me to discover just how many unnatural and chemical-filled ingredients were in the food I'd been buying. As anxious and overwhelmed as I felt after leaving his office, I was determined to do whatever it took to help my daughter. Feeding Kaleigh became a full-time job. Eating outside the home was almost impossible, so we brought Kaleigh's food everywhere we went. She couldn't eat what was served at holiday events or birthday parties, since her diet was now mostly whole organic foods. Looking back, I realize how naive I was about our food system. If it was on the supermarket shelf, I'd assumed, it was safe to feed my family. What I began to discover was quite disturbing.

Over the past few decades, nothing may have changed more drastically than the way we grow, process, and eat food in the United States. Some of the changes have been positive and include advancements in convenience items, food and allergy labeling, and a focus on more healthful, natural, and organic food choices. However, despite many of our advancements, as a country we still have a long way to go with many of our food protocols.

Unless we awaken to the reality that many of the newer practices within our food system are causing harm, we won't be able to make improvements in the health and well-being of our children. In other words, we can't fix a problem we don't know exists. So, in this chapter we will take a closer look at some of the major changes to our food system over the past few decades. First, we will briefly discuss *processed food* choices, and then examine the major changes that have occurred in our *whole food* choices as well. We will take a closer look at how new farming practices have greatly impacted the final food products we serve our families and how food can play a key role in both identifying and treating some of our children's health problems.

Section 1: Processed Food

I'm not sure what makes pepperoni so good—if it's the pepper or the oni.
—S. A. Sachs

Most of us already know that processed foods are not always the healthiest. Unfortunately, given the reality of our fast-paced lives, the nutritional value of a meal is often sacrificed for what's quick and convenient. Fifty years ago, our grandparents ate real food, but today, most of the food we offer our children is nutritionally depleted and made with artificial ingredients linked to a host of medical disorders. Chemicals have been steadily infiltrating our food system since the 1950s. They are used to add shelf life, texture, color, and flavor, but may also promote chronic disease in the human body.

In the United States there are over 3,000 food additives approved for use. Whether or not they're safe for long-term consumption or in combination with each other is a troubling question. Other countries, many in Europe, employ the precautionary principle that requires a manufacturer to prove a food additive is safe before it's permitted on store shelves. However, here in the United States, the FDA needs to prove that a food additive is dangerous to get it *off* store shelves—because that's the law according to Congress. This system contains enormous loopholes that allow additives of questionable safety to be listed as "Generally Recognized as Safe" or GRAS. Let's take a closer look at just one food additive that other countries have regulated—artificial food coloring, or food dyes.

Health Impacts of Food Dyes

In the United States, adding artificial coloring, or dye, to processed food is common practice. Studies have shown that these additives can have a harmful effect on our children's health. Many of the dyes have been linked to behavioral problems in children, and some have even been linked to cancer. Concerns about food coloring have been around since the 1970s, and since then many countries have addressed the issue with outright bans on suspect dyes, or special labeling requirements on products that contain them. The European Union now requires warning labels on food containing specific dyes. These labels spell out to consumers that the food product they are purchasing may have an adverse effect on the activity and attention of children. The British government took additional action, and now food manufacturers in the United Kingdom are removing most synthetic dyes from the foods sold there. Yet, here in the United States, food manufacturers are *not* required to specially label products that contain these same additives. Should they be? We hardly think it's a coincidence that as we've increased the amount of food dyes we consume in America, the number of children diagnosed with conditions such as ADD and ADHD has also increased. Adopting the same warning labels that other countries have in place would let parents make more informed decisions. The following graph highlights the problem.

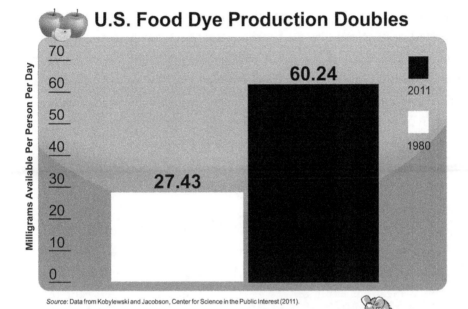

U.S. Food Dye Production Doubles

Milligrams Available Per Person Per Day

70
60
50
40
30
20
10
0

60.24

2011

1980

27.43

Source: Data from Kobylewski and Jacobson, Center for Science in the Public Interest (2011).

⇨ According to the Center for Science in the Public Interest (CSPI), numerous studies have been published that shed light on how a child's diet can have adverse effects on their behavior and strongly suggest an association between ingestion of synthetic food dyes and hyperactivity that reverses when the dyes are removed.

⇨ Food colorings (Blue 1, Blue 2, Citrus Red 2, Green 3, Red 3, Red 40, Yellow 5, and Yellow 6) can be found in all kinds of children's snacks, candy, colored drinks, cereal, vitamins, medications, and more (including medications for ADD/ADHD).

⇨ According to CSPI, the three most widely used dyes, Red 40, Yellow 5, and Yellow 6 are also contaminated with known carcinogens (chemicals known to cause cancer) and Blue 1, Blue 2, and Green 3 have been shown to cause cancer in animals.

⇨ Additionally, Red 3 has been acknowledged for years by the FDA to be a carcinogen. The FDA has banned it from cosmetics and externally applied drugs. However, it still remains in our ingested drugs and our food supply due to pressure from the food industry at the time the initial ban was proposed.

⇨ Most artificial food colorings also contain small amounts of mercury, lead, and arsenic.

Encouraging News about Food Dyes

Many different studies and personal accounts from parents show how simple elimination diets can reverse hyperactivity and behavioral problems when food dyes are suspected. And some retailers, such as Whole Foods, have made this elimination easier for parents by banning artificial food dyes, along with other questionable ingredients, from their stores. For more information on food dyes, including many published studies, visit the website of the Center for Science in the Public Interest. Our Resource Guide in Part 3 or at www.behindcloseddoorsthebook.com provides more detailed information.

FINDING FOCUS (CATHY, FIFTH-GRADE TEACHER)

One of my students had hyperactivity, trouble focusing, and anger issues from an early age. While conferencing with his mom, the topic of medications came up. As a parent myself, I wouldn't want my child to endure medication unless deemed totally necessary due to the many associated side effects. So I broached the subject of diet and shared all I had learned about the health effects of food dyes. I find that many parents are aware of the impacts of sugar in a child's diet but less aware of the possible effects of food coloring. I shared an experience with another child that had many of the same behavioral problems this conferencing mom was facing, and the family eventually found the culprit was red food dye used in the drinks the child consumed daily. The mom I was conferencing with thanked me for sharing the story and thought eliminating food dyes (especially red) was definitely worth a try. Within a week of altering her son's diet, I witnessed a profound effect on her son's behaviors and socialization in the classroom. His mother reported the same positive changes at home and later told me he was even able to focus enough to learn music, which provided an outlet for his creativity and a big boost to his self-esteem.

How Does Our Processed Food Compare with Other Countries'?

Because many of the food additives permitted in the United States have been banned in other countries, often due to possible health effects, manufacturers make different versions of their products to meet each nation's regulatory requirements. This means that a company will eliminate a known health hazard from a product it sells to one country but continue to put that same dangerous additive in the product sold in the United States. For example, Kellogg's Nutri-Grain bars sold in Great Britain are made with natural colorings (beetroot red, annatto, paprika), but when sold in the United States they're made with food dyes (red no. 40, yellow no. 6, blue no. 1)—all linked to behavioral problems in children.

Other common food additives used in the United States and banned in other countries include BHA, BHT, synthetic hormones (rBGH and rBST), olestra, azodicarbonamide, and arsenic. If you see any of the banned ingredients just mentioned on your food labels, you may want to think twice about your purchase. More information on these banned ingredients can be found in the Resource Guide in Part 3 or at www.behindcloseddoorsthebook.com. If healthier versions of our food are available from manufacturers for consumers in other countries, shouldn't they be made available to U.S. consumers too? Processed foods may very well play a big role in the chronic health problems our children are experiencing.

NOT ONE HAND [LIZ]

Christine and I have been good friends for the past ten years and she knew that I had volunteered to host an international exchange student from Spain. When she called to see how it was going I shared with her that the group of fifty Spanish high school students had planned to get together for group dinners with their host families throughout their time in the United States. One of the organizing mothers stood up in front of the exchange students and asked, "How many of you have food allergies or sensitivities we need to take into consideration when planning meals?" The kids from Spain all looked bewildered by the question and not one hand went up.

Did You Know?

It wasn't until 1990 that packaged foods were required to bear nutrition labeling under the Nutrition Labeling and Education Act.

Processed Food Practical Tools

It's important to note that not all food additives pose health risks; in fact, many food additives are safe. In the Resource Guide (see in Part 3 or www. behindcloseddoorsthebook.com), we've provided a list of food additives experts find to be safe and a list of food additives experts feel we should avoid. We've also included an eye-opening food infographic, courtesy of the *Center for Science in the Public Interest,* showing the process the FDA uses for companies to get a chemical food additive approved.

Most of us will never have the time to look into every single ingredient on our food labels. The Resource Guide (see Part 3 or www.behindcloseddoors thebook.com) contains great time-saving solutions to help you make healthier food choices, including online resources that provide *safety ratings* on thousands of food items found in the grocery store. They offer databases by food product or individual ingredient and some even provide smart phone apps so you can simply scan a UPC code and get product information sent right to your phone while shopping. One of our favorites is *The Good Guide* (more details on this tool and others can be found in the Resource Guide).

Section 2: Genetically Modified Foods

The major problems in the world are the result of the difference between how nature works and the way people think.
—Gregory Bateson

One of the biggest and most controversial changes to our food supply over the past twenty-five years has been the adoption of genetically modified foods. Such foods are often referred to as GMOs (genetically modified organisms). The story behind GMOs reveals how consumer protection has taken a backseat to industry influences, and how this new food practice may prove to be a big player in many of the chronic illnesses we're seeing on the rise in our children.

GMOs have infiltrated both our processed food *and* our whole food choices. Many of us are well aware of the growth and expansion of processed foods over the years. This is obvious because they take up the majority of shelf space in the average grocery store. Most of us are probably less aware of the major changes that have occurred in our *whole food* choices as well. Whole foods are unprocessed, unrefined, and grown or raised in nature. Examples include vegetables, fruits, whole grains, and animal products.

There is no more appropriate place to start a discussion of the changes within our whole foods than with the American farmer. After all, it is the American farmer that raises the livestock that produce our dairy and meat products. It is the American farmer that cultivates the land and plants the seeds for our vegetables, fruit, and commodity crops. Until recently, the American farmer was the one trusted person standing behind most source ingredients of our food, whole or processed. Because farming has gone through so many changes over the past few decades, the farmer has become less involved in how animals are raised and crops are grown. Major food companies, who contract with farmers, are the ones often calling the shots on many U.S. farms today and clearly influencing the final products we buy and serve to our children. We will explore the changes to our whole foods in three sections, starting here with the adoption of genetically modified food, followed by the movement from conventional farming to industrialized farming, and finally how these influences have impacted American farmers.

FOOD MATTERS (KRISTIE, MOMS ACROSS AMERICA)

One day I stopped at the doctor's office to get my daughter Caroline's nut allergy information signed for school. They weren't able to complete the paperwork (or refill her Epi-pen) because she hadn't been in for a visit in twenty months. My first reaction was to get angry and then I took a minute to let that sink in . . . TWENTY MONTHS. My girl with asthma, eczema, chronic pneumonia, food allergies, and hip dysplasia hasn't been to the doctor in almost two years! Is it a coincidence that we changed how we eat (to non-GMO and organic) almost two years ago? I think not! She's living proof that the foods we eat and the products we put on our bodies matter.

If you have never heard of GMOs, you're not alone. Surveys show that only about one in every four Americans know they've been eating foods derived from genetically modified crops since they were approved for use in the mid-1990s. GMOs have been banned or require labeling in sixty-four other countries, including the entire European Union. Yet in the United States, there are no clear federal labeling requirements for these foods. This is a critical topic in desperate need of more transparency in our country.

What Are GMOs?

GMOs are the result of a laboratory process in which scientists extract genes (pieces of DNA) from one plant or animal and artificially transfer the genes into another plant or animal. The foreign genes may come from bacteria, viruses, insects, animals, or plants, and the process allows genes to be transferred *across* natural species. For example, a specific animal trait is inserted into a plant or vice versa. By successfully inserting jellyfish genes into potatoes, scientists have tested the ability to create potatoes that glow in the dark when they need watering.

It's absolutely impossible for this process to happen naturally, and it is not yet an exact science. This science is being carried out by biotech companies, many of whom got their start as *chemical* companies, bringing us products like PCBs, bovine growth hormone, Agent Orange, and DDT. These chemical companies are now fundamentally involved in the world's food supply. The technology they're developing is most commonly marketed in the form of a genetically modified *seed* that's patented and sold to farmers who grow our crops. The most common genetically modified crops in the United States are corn, followed by soy and cottonseed.

Why Are Foods Genetically Modified?

These products are most frequently genetically modified to *withstand* large amounts of pesticides (both herbicides and insecticides). It goes without saying that pesticide use on our food crops raises serious health concerns, especially for infants and children because of their potential for toxicity.

One specific crop is being genetically modified to withstand higher than natural amounts of *herbicides* (weed killers—such as Roundup) without the crops dying as they normally would from the toxicity. These are known as HT (herbicide-tolerant) crops, and varieties may include corn, soy, cotton, canola, sugar beets, and alfalfa.

Crops are also being genetically modified to produce their own internal insecticide, a Bt (Bacillus thuringiensis) toxin, that targets and kill pests that may try to eat the crops. These genetically modified crops are known as Bt crops and varieties may include corn and cotton. Although these crops were marketed with the promise of less *external* pesticide use, insecticides are still part of the equation and part of the food itself, with every cell of the plant we eat secreting the insecticidal toxin.

In short, new and unnatural gene traits are being incorporated into the existing DNA of food crops through the development of genetically modified seeds sold to farmers who plant and grow our food. These two crop varieties (HT and Bt) currently produce the majority of GMO foods in the United States. Do we want our children eating food products derived from crops producing their own insecticide? Or crops that now have the ability to survive an otherwise deadly dose of a toxic weed killer like Roundup and its main ingredient glyphosate? How will these pesticides affect a developing nervous system? Food derived from these specialty crops are being sold *without* any clear labeling requirements so we won't know if the foods we purchase and feed our families contain them. Many find this concerning.

Did You Know?

The International Agency for Research on Cancer (IARC), the specialized agency of the World Health Organization, has classified *glyphosate*, the main ingredient in Roundup and widely used on genetically modified crops, as probably *carcinogenic* to humans. The IARC also concluded that glyphosate can cause DNA and chromosomal damage in human cells.

According to a 2014 article by Dr. Ramon J. Seidler, a former EPA senior scientist, published in the Environmental Working Group's online "AgMag," the increased presence of pesticides (herbicides, insecticides, and fungicides) as a result of genetically modified HT and Bt crops is a growing problem. By 2010, these crops began to show the emergence of pesticide-resistant weeds and insects, requiring additional pesticides to combat the problem. The USDA has reported that since 1996, glyphosate use has increased about twelve-fold. These toxic pesticides not only contaminate our food and water, but also increase our body burden of chemicals and pose significant risks to the nervous and endocrine systems of developing infants and children. Dr. Seidler points out that the growing problem provides an all-too-convenient opportunity for additional profits for the chemical companies that developed and sold the seeds to the farmers in the first place. Now they can offer farmers *additional* chemicals and *additional* genetically modified seeds to combat the problem.

Are GMO Foods Tested and Safe?

Unlike safety testing required for a new drug in the United States, no laws demand premarket safety testing for GMO foods. The FDA *believes* foods derived from genetically modified crops are no different than foods derived from their conventional non-GMO crop counterparts. The FDA's own scientists and doctors initially warned that GMO foods could result in toxicity problems, unpredictable risks such as hidden allergens, and the potential to accelerate the spread of antibiotic-resistant disease. But GMOs were fast-tracked despite these concerns. The FDA has never declared GMO foods to be safe for human consumption. Instead, it says that the food producers who make them believe that they're safe for humans.

The FDA approval process currently allows for safety assessments to be conducted by the companies seeking approval of their genetically modified food crop. *Let's repeat that one.* Safety assessments are conducted by the very companies seeking approval. Does their obvious vested financial interest in the outcome of their own safety evaluations allow for a fair and balanced process? To make matters worse, these safety studies aren't made available for public review or any type of peer-reviewed publication because companies feel that sharing the information may infringe on the intellectual property rights of the GMO food crops (genetically modified seeds are patented and owned by the biotech companies). So there is no transparency in the approval process, which in turn cannot ensure food safety for our children.

The bottom line is that GMOs have completely infiltrated our food system without adequate safety studies to understand the full impacts on human health— let alone the health of our children. And the biotech companies controlling the crops and the manufacturers selling GMO foods continually block food labeling efforts. The obvious question is, "If GMO foods are so safe and beneficial, then why do these industries spend millions of dollars in political lobbying efforts to keep GMO labels *off* their products and consumers in the dark?"

GMO Studies and Our Children's Health

Because children's bodies are smaller and growing at a faster pace than adults', they're more likely to experience the possible health effects of GMO foods. Additionally, more than half of our immune system resides in and near the digestive tract, making any damaging effects from food a possible factor in many conditions, but especially those that are autoimmune in nature.

As we've noted, foods derived from genetically modified crops may contain chemical pesticides that pose significant risks to the nervous and endocrine systems of developing infants and children. Peer-reviewed studies have found that genetically modified foods can have unintended toxic and allergenic effects, as well as an altered nutritional value. Below are some specific concerns from

GMO feeding studies in laboratory and farm animals, as well as from studies on pesticides related to genetically modified crops.

- Animal feeding studies indicate that GMO foods may be associated with allergic reactions, infertility, damaged immune systems, impaired digestive function, and damage to most organ and body systems studied in animals.
- Toxic effects of glyphosate found in animal and in vitro experiments include disruption of hormonal systems and beneficial gut bacteria, developmental and reproductive toxicity, malformations, cancer, and neurotoxicity.

These studies show potential problems from GMO food consumption and indicate a strong need for additional research. As mothers, we feel that we've reached a breaking point in our current food system. Without any independent safety testing required for GMO food approvals, who will look out for the health and safety of our children? We don't think it's a coincidence that many of the same health problems exhibited in lab animals and livestock fed GMO foods are also on the rise in U.S. children. For instance, studies showed that animals fed GMO corn exhibited an increased appetite, weight gain, and suffered stomach and digestive problems as well as immune system problems. Is it possible, if not likely, that GMO corn and its association with glyphosate have contributed to the rise of obesity and autoimmune disorders such as food allergies and inflammatory bowel disease in children since it was introduced in 1996?

One recent *human* study, published in 2011 by the *Journal of Reproductive Toxicology*, sheds light on how this change in our food system may already be affecting our children's health and demonstrates just how lax our country's GMO food approval process has been. The biotech companies originally claimed that the insecticidal protein (Bt) in some GM plants would be broken down in the digestive tract and unable to get into blood or body tissues to cause toxic effects. This claim was shown to be false by several studies, including the one in the *Journal of Reproductive Toxicology*. Bt wasn't destroyed in the stomach, but was very capable of being passed through the umbilical cord from a mother to her unborn baby—as Bt was found in 93 percent of the mothers and 80 percent of the unborn babies tested. If this industry assumption was incorrect, how many other ones will also prove to be wrong?

The American Academy of Environmental Medicine (AAEM) has found "more than a casual relationship between GMO foods and adverse health effects." They believe there is ample evidence of probable harm and that it's imperative to adopt precautionary principles when it comes to GMO foods. The AAEM recommends avoiding GMO foods when possible and asks physicians to consider the possible role of GMO foods in the disease process of patients they treat. The organization has called for a moratorium on GMO food, implementation of immediate long-term independent safety testing, and labeling of GMO foods, all deemed necessary for the health and safety of consumers.

What Foods Contain GMOs?

GMO corn, soy, canola, and sugar beets are most commonly used to produce raw ingredients for our processed food. They're widely found in foods such as vegetable oils, snacks, breakfast cereal, soft drinks, and margarine. About *80 percent of our processed foods contain GMO ingredients*, so any food ingredients derived from corn, soy, canola, and sugar beets may possibly contain GMOs. Corn is by far the most widespread GMO product and would be a good starting point for those choosing to avoid GMO ingredients. High-fructose corn syrup, which has broadly infiltrated our food system, is highly derived from GMO corn.

GMO foods have expanded well beyond the aforementioned crops. Salmon genetically modified with a growth hormone (to grow twice as big and twice as fast) has recently been approved by the FDA. Additionally, much of the milk in the United States comes from cows that could potentially be injected with a genetically modified growth hormone. And other GMO foods, such as genetically modified apples (that don't turn brown when cut open) and genetically modified potatoes (that won't bruise) are already far along the FDA approval process and may soon be available as *whole foods* at your local grocery store. All of these GMO foods are being sold in grocery stores every day—with no clear labeling requirements.

REMOVING THE REASON (KAREN, MOMS ACROSS AMERICA)

My seven-year-old old son was diagnosed with asthma and needed glasses inside of two weeks of that diagnosis. I started learning about asthma and natural ways to control it, but then I found out about GMOs. Once I removed my family from GMO foods/drinks my son went from needing a nebulizer three times a day to not at all. His asthma disappeared and he no longer had the astigmatism that required glasses. The eye doctor said he must have had "some sort of inflammation" that was now gone for whatever reason. The reason was removing GMOs from our diets. Last year, my son was recommended for retention. This year he's at the top of his class.

The chart below may help you visualize just how rapidly the United States has adopted GMO food crops.

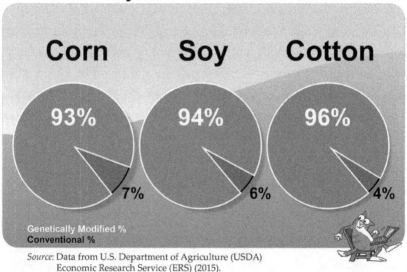

Total Percent of U.S. Crops
Genetically Modified vs. Conventional

Corn   **Soy**   **Cotton**

93%   94%   96%

7%   6%   4%

Genetically Modified %
Conventional %

Source: Data from U.S. Department of Agriculture (USDA)
Economic Research Service (ERS) (2015).

The quick adoption of genetically modified crops has led to fewer and fewer conventional (non-GMO) crops being planted in our country. But as more and more consumers become aware of GMOs in our food and consider the environmental, health, and social consequences of the industrialized food production, demand for non-GMO foods and foods raised more sustainably and/or organically has risen. As a result, some farmers are beginning to revert back to traditional crop varieties.

Currently, there are sixty-four nations that require labeling of GMO food or have outright banned GMO foods. Other governments are taking a stance to protect their citizens and the environment from the potential health impacts of GMOs. In the United States, the FDA declares GMOs to be essentially no different than conventional food. According to many recent polls, over 90 percent of Americans believe they have the right to know about the foods they eat and feed their families—a basic right that citizens in other parts of the world have secured through mandatory GMO labeling laws.

By 2016, Vermont, Connecticut, Maine, and Virginia had all passed GMO labeling laws and more than half of all U.S. states introduced bills for clear GMO labeling or outright bans. However, later that year, President Obama passed an industry friendly federal GMO labeling law that overturned these state laws and completely undermined our right to know what is in our food. Contrary to what you would think would be required for a federal GMO labeling law, it does not require food manufacturers to label GMO food clearly. For example, it is acceptable for a product bar code to be our labeling—requiring us to scan a food product using a smart phone app to see if it contains GMO ingredients! Does this new law represent what most Americans wanted or what the industry wanted? Here is the good news, despite the food industries influence on politics, consumers are still winning. Manufacturers are realizing that consumers want to know if the product they are buying contain GMO ingredients and are voluntarily labeling their product as non-GMO. More information on labeling efforts and ways to get involved are found in the Resource Guide in Part 3 or at www.behindcloseddoorsthebook.com.

Encouraging News about GMOs

- Cheerios cereal is a popular snack for many babies and toddlers in the United States. In Europe, children have been enjoying non-GMO

Cheerios for quite some time. Due to pressure from activist groups and consumers, in 2014 General Mills announced that they've stopped using GMO ingredients to make original Cheerios cereal sold in the United States. *[Authors' note: GMO ingredients are still in other flavors of Cheerios sold in the United States.]*

- Many across the food and restaurant industry are also beginning to start non-GMO efforts. In 2015, Chipotle Mexican Grill became the first national restaurant chain to be GMO-free. This new standard will increase pressure for many in the restaurant business to start to find suppliers that do not use genetically modified crops.

- Whole Foods Market announced that by 2018 it would require labeling of genetically engineered foods sold in its stores—a big victory for consumers.

- Moms Across America is a growing grassroots organization of moms educating the public about the dangers of GMOs and pesticides. (We're grateful for their permission to include Kristie and Karen's stories, above.) Their website includes video interviews with doctors concerned about the health risks of GMOs and some great testimonials from mothers about the health improvements their children experien becoming GMO free. More information is in the Resource Guide in Part 3 or at www.behindcloseddoorsthebook.com.

GMO Practical Tools

The most powerful way to protect our children until clear consumer labeling is required in America is through buying less processed and packaged food. We can also ensure our food contains no GMOs by purchasing food certified with the *Non-GMO Project seal* (look for the butterfly) or *certified organic food* (the certification prohibits the use of any GMO ingredients).

See the Resource Guide for additional information on current GMO labeling laws, common foods that contain GMOs, and how to obtain a Non-GMO Shopping Guide (courtesy of the Non-GMO Project and the Institute for Responsible Technology).

Section 3: Industrialized Farming

The measure of a society can be how well its people treat its animals.
—Mohandas Gandhi

OPENING EYES (CHRISTINE)

While attending a parent-teacher conference a few years ago, I expressed my gratitude to the teacher for being so vigilant in helping to maintain a safe school environment for Kaleigh's food allergies. The teacher told me that the school district was considering a ban on all foods for school parties and activities because so many children had food allergies. He shook his head and said he couldn't fathom what was causing this. When I shared with him what I'd been learning about our broken food system, his eyes widened and then he nodded in agreement when I said the epidemic of food allergies is likely no coincidence.

Let's turn to the next changed practice affecting our whole foods—the move from conventional farming to industrialized farming. Exploring this change will allow us to see how this newer farming practice may just cut straight to the heart of many of our nation's health problems. Our discussion will also demonstrate how the U.S. food industry has become the powerful trillion-dollar-a-year business it is today.

Industrialized farming often focuses on one type of crop production or one type of animal raised for food (known as monoculture farming). Industrialized farming is also sometimes referred to as factory farming because unlike traditional farming practices, factory farms attempt to maximize food production while minimizing costs. To do this, they often operate without proper consideration of animal health, environmental health, workers' health, or consumer health. This is the way most meat, dairy, eggs, fruit, and vegetables are now produced and delivered to our supermarkets. These are our whole foods, which should be the most nutritious and healthy food options we have.

One of the best alternative methods to industrialized farming is *sustainable farming*. According to Sustainable Table, a leading sustainable food resource for consumers, sustainable agriculture is the production of food using farming methods that protect the health and welfare of animals, humans, the environment, and communities. It aims to produce healthful food without compromising a future generation's ability to do the same. A sustainable farmer relies on symbiotic relationships with nature and renewable resources, instead of synthetic pesticides, artificial hormones, or the routine use of antibiotics. Sustainable farming is a way of farming or a set of farming principles. It's not a certification such as "organic"; while many sustainable farms have organic certifications, the terms are not interchangeable.

Let's take a deeper look at what's really happening with our food. Pictures can help us understand the different practices behind the food labels at the grocery store. They also serve to provide us with some reassurance that we always have *choices* when it comes to the food products we consume. We'll examine both our industrial and sustainable farming choices by viewing how our fruits, vegetables, grains, meats, and dairy are grown or raised under each farming method. This will allow us to see more clearly how our daily food choices can influence our children's health.

Industrialized Agriculture: Fruits, Vegetables, and Grains from Monocrops

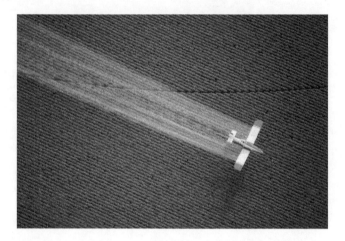

- Industrialized crops often rely on the technology of genetically modified seeds.
- Growing a single crop over a large amount of land requires more chemical fertilizers, pesticides, herbicides, and fungicides. It can also cause the soil to be overworked and lose nutrients.
- Chemical inputs can be damaging to the environment, communities, and farm workers.
- Exposure to pesticides is especially dangerous to infants and children: not only does it increase the risk of developing cancer, but it can also negatively affect the nervous system, immune system, and reproductive system.
- Increased chemicals in crops = increased chemicals in our food = increased chemicals in our children's bodies and our own.

Sustainable Agriculture: Fruits, Vegetables, and Grains from Diversified Crops

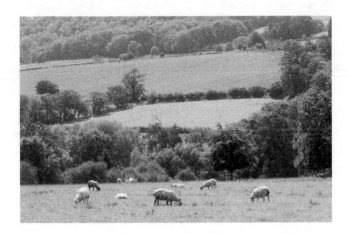

- Genetically modified seeds are not used in sustainable farming (and are prohibited in organic farming).
- Planting multiple crops reduces the need for chemical pesticides, herbicides, and fungicides (organic certification completely prohibits these chemical inputs).
- Sustainable farming practices minimize fossil fuel consumption and protect the soil from loss of critical nutrients.
- Less chemicals in our crops = less chemicals in our food = less chemicals in our children's bodies.
- Healthy soil = nutrient-dense food = more nutrients in our children's bodies.

911 OATMEAL (CHRISTINE)

When Kaleigh was three years old, she loved to help in the kitchen. Being under my constant supervision, she'd grown accustomed to understanding what foods she could and could not have. One day when my mom was watching her, she wanted to help make oatmeal. Although she knew she couldn't have this kind of oatmeal (due to her gluten sensitivity), she still wanted to help make breakfast for Grandmom. As she was opening the packet of oatmeal she inhaled some of the dust released as she poured it into the bowl. As a result of simply breathing it in, her face and tongue began to swell and she developed hives. My mom reacted quickly giving her Benadryl and then called 911. I met the ambulance at the hospital and in a few hours Kaleigh's reaction began to subside and we were able to return home. This was not the first 911 call and, unfortunately, not the last.

Industrialized vs. Sustainable Livestock

Until recently, livestock (animals raised for food or other products) were naturally integrated with crop production on a farm and raised in a balanced way beneficial to both the farmers and the animals. But in the last few decades livestock production has undergone a transformation. Animals have been moved off pastures and are now being raised indoors, held in large feeding areas known as CAFOs (confined animal feeding operations). In this setting, production and profits can be maximized. CAFOs are characterized by large numbers of animals crowded into tight spaces, an unnatural and unhealthy situation for both animals and workers. CAFOs now dominate the U.S. meat and dairy industry and represent the common practice behind most meat and dairy foods commercially available.

According to Sustainable Table, "truly sustainable livestock farming requires the use of a pasture-based system." When animals are raised on pasture, they can roam freely in their natural environment and carry out their natural behaviors. They can also graze on nutritious grasses and other plant foods found in nature that their bodies are adapted to digest. Let's compare how a chicken is raised using sustainable farming vs. industrialized factory farming. After viewing this one example, decide for yourself if the way an animal is raised impacts the quality of food we ultimately feed our families.

Did You Know?

Medication containing *arsenic* is often added to the feed of chickens raised for food to stimulate growth, reduce infections, and make the flesh an appetizing shade of pink. The EPA classifies inorganic arsenic as a human *carcinogen*.

Chicken from Factory Farms

- Broiler (meat) chickens typically spend their lives in stress and confined to warehouse-type sheds, with little or no natural light, and no access to the outdoors.

- Sheds are packed with as many as 20,000 chickens, leaving little if any room for natural movements such as spreading their wings. On average, the space for each chicken is about one square foot.

- Floors of the sheds can be covered in the waste of tens of thousands of chickens creating excessive ammonia levels. The overwhelming stench causes breathing difficulties and other health problems for both chickens and workers.

- The artificial lights in the sheds are on almost constantly to stimulate eating and unnaturally rapid growth of the chickens.

- Chickens are routinely fed low-cost feed that often includes genetically modified corn and soy. Other feed additives may include animal byproducts, antibiotics, and other medications.

- Chickens have been subjected to intense genetic selection to produce chickens with bigger breasts and thighs in the shortest period of time so that chickens can reach market weight in only six or seven weeks—half the time it took in the 1950s.

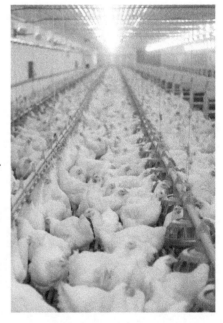

- At six weeks, many broiler chickens have such large and heavy breasts that they have difficulty supporting their own body weight and spend much of their time lying down.

- There is no law requiring chickens (or turkeys or any birds) to be rendered unconscious before slaughter, and as a result they often needlessly suffer.

Chicken from Sustainable Farms

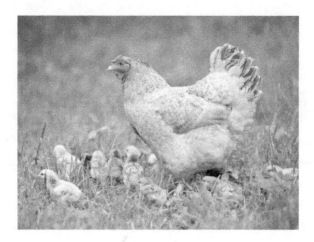

- Chickens have access to pasture on a regular basis where they can roam freely through the grass, get fresh air and sunshine, and enjoy rooting, pecking, and digging for worms and other natural food.
- Chickens are always free to carry out their natural behaviors and will enjoy a diet free of any unnatural feed additives. They may also actively forage on pasture, which provides supplemental nutrients.
- Organic chickens must be fed only 100 percent certified organic feed, grown without artificial fertilizers or pesticides. The pastures they roam must also be 100 percent organic and antibiotics are prohibited.
- Sustainable farmers only raise as many chickens as their land can responsibly support. They also avoid chemical pesticides and raise chickens without routine use of antibiotics.
- Sustainable chickens must be raised in a way that nurtures the ecology of the entire farm, including the health of the pasture, proper waste disposal, conservation of resources, and the maintenance of all vegetation and wildlife on the farm.

Conscious Eating

*The power of a movement lies in the fact
that it can indeed change the habits of people.*
—Steve Biko

The reality behind some of our industrialized food practices may have shocked and upset you—especially if you are learning about them for the first time. Many of our current food practices are quite disturbing and in desperate need of reform. We need to return to more humane and sustainable practices, while questioning the ethics behind factory farming operations and the way we treat animals raised for food. When we consume food derived from animals raised in unhealthy conditions, we will undoubtedly experience its negative health effects.

The good news is that you've now viewed some solutions to these problems. Sustainable farmers use much more ethical practices, properly feeding and caring for their livestock in healthy, humane, and responsible ways. These holistic practices must become the norm again if we wish to see healthy children and a thriving environment. Although food is just one of the issues affecting our children's health, it may be the most important, as it is a critical component of our overall well-being. It is what sustains us, gives us vital life force, and enables our bodies to function. We'll talk about more specific solutions in the Practical Tools section below.

The Impacts of Industrial Farming

*The rise in animal factories over the last fifty years has led to a
system that is out of control. Mad cow disease, increased liver
abscesses, and the rise of antibiotic-resistant bacteria are just
some examples of the damage that comes from unwise and
often inhumane approaches to raising food animals.*
—The Union of Concerned Scientists

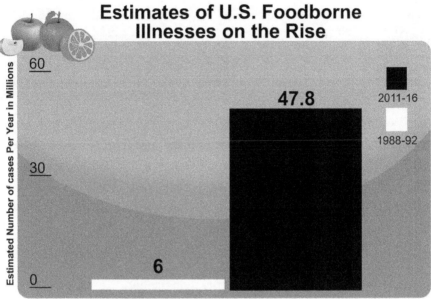

Estimates of U.S. Foodborne Illnesses on the Rise

47.8

2011-16

1988-92

6

Estimated Number of cases Per Year in Millions

60

30

0

Includes Estimates of Both Known and Unknown Agents

Sources: 1988-92 data from Bean, *CDC Morbidity and Mortality Weekly Report (MMWR)* (1996). 2011 data from Scallan, *Emerging Infectious Diseases* (2011). 2016 data from the Centers for Disease Control and Prevention (CDC) (2016).
Note: In October 1999 the CDC revised their Foodborne Disease Outbreak Surveillance System (FBDOSS); as a result data from 1990 cannot be directly compared to data from 2011 due to changes in methods of data collection. In 2016, the CDC estimates remained 47.8 cases a year.

▷ When we changed from traditional farming and agriculture practices to an industrialized style of farming and agriculture did we manufacture more foodborne illnesses?

▷ According to the World Health Organization (WHO), changed farming practices and industrialized factory farming food production may have led to the emergence of new animal diseases that affect humans.

▷ It's not just agriculture contributing, seafood products cause about 20% of the known outbreaks of foodborne illnesses each year.

▷ Those at greatest risk for harmful effects from foodborne illnesses are infants and children, pregnant women and their unborn babies, older adults, and people with weakened immune systems.

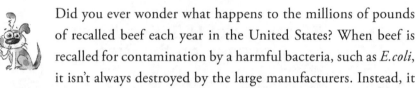

Did You Know?

Did you ever wonder what happens to the millions of pounds of recalled beef each year in the United States? When beef is recalled for contamination by a harmful bacteria, such as *E.coli*, it isn't always destroyed by the large manufacturers. Instead, it often ends up for sale again on the supermarket shelves in canned goods that contain cooked beef and frozen packaged products with cooked beef. According to the USDA's Food Safety and Inspection Service, beef that is recalled due to contamination can be "restored to wholesomeness after it is fully cooked to full lethality [i.e., a dose of heat high enough to kill the bacteria]." No special labeling is required because that *would* be bad for business, wouldn't it? The same concept applies to poultry.

THE COST OF HEALTHY FOOD (JOANNE)

I met a mother of three at a baby shower and we began talking about her kids. They had many of the typical health problems we had all grown accustom to hearing about: ADD, allergies, and gastrointestinal issues. The mother told me about how all the medications and tests for these chronic illnesses—as well as her own—were taking a financial toll on her family. Both she and her husband worked full-time, but they could barely keep up with the medical bills. Other moms joined in our conversation, and we all began offering various suggestions that had worked for our children. When we talked about avoiding processed foods and trying to eat organic, non-GMO foods the mother chuckled and said, "Are you kidding? I'd love to be able to feed my children those types of foods. But the truth is, we simply can't afford it."

A large part of our health-related food problem stems from economics. Processed foods are often cheaper than whole foods. A major factor behind this price disparity are government subsidies for farmers who produce large monocrops (especially corn), which we all pay for in tax dollars. This subsidized corn drives our factory farms (as genetically modified animal feed) and drives our processed foods (as high fructose corn syrup), making soft drinks and snack foods with empty calories much more affordable than nutrient-dense, sustainably grown whole foods.

When we begin to understand the types of foods that are truly affordable and available to the 22 percent of American children living in poverty, we see why these same children are often most riddled with chronic disease and childhood obesity. If we want to improve the health of our children, we need to make healthy food more affordable and accessible for everyone. Wouldn't it make more sense to take all those corn subsidies supporting our industrialized food system and transfer them to subsidies for sustainably grown fruits and vegetables? We need to restructure our agricultural policies so that they can better promote health and sustainability for *all* children.

Sustainable Farming Practical Tools

Thankfully, the sustainable food movement, often supported by the small American farmer, is emerging and growing rapidly across our country. The Resource Guide (see Part 3 or www.behindcloseddoorsthebook.com) provides you with information from the Sustainable Table to help you easily locate farmers in your local area who offer foods raised sustainably. They also offer information on organic agriculture.

We also included information on *seafood* as a supplement in the Resource Guide. Here you can review how the same concept of factory farming animals applies to our seafood and find helpful health information. You'll find a sample *fish guide* courtesy of the Environmental Defense Fund, which can help you avoid dangerous levels of harmful contaminants present in seafood (such as mercury and the chemical PCB) based on a person's age and gender. Additional information is available regarding government fish guides and advisories.

Section 4: The Plight of the American Farmer

*Good farmers, who take seriously their duties as stewards of Creation and
of their land's inheritors, contribute to the welfare of society in more ways
than society usually acknowledges, or even knows.*
—Wendell Berry

Over the past few decades, the American farmer has endured many struggles that have essentially changed our food system. Prior to the industrial revolution, approximately one in every four Americans worked in some aspect of farming. Today only 2 percent of Americans work in farming, so where did all the U.S. farmers go? The answer sums up all that's changed in our food practices and exposes the corrosive stronghold of political and economic influences throughout our culture.

In the early 1970s, the U.S. government more or less asked farmers to "get big or get out." They began to provide large subsidies (financial support) to agribusinesses that supported *monocultures* (farming one type of product, such as corn). This type of farming maximized crop yields and profitability, which supported a political and economic agenda set up for our *industrialized* food system. Many farmers decided to "get big" and remained. But many small, independent or diversified farmers were forced to "get out" because they couldn't compete with the lower prices larger, subsidized farmers could now offer the food industry.

Through mergers and acquisitions, big companies also began to control many different levels of the food supply chain. The end result was consolidation, with fewer farms producing the raw ingredients for our food products and fewer companies offering to buy from the remaining farmers. Currently, behind the wide variety of company labels that fill the grocery stores are only a handful of large corporations that own a good portion of the labels. They dominate most aspects of the food system and have enormous power to control markets and pricing and to influence food and agriculture regulations. They can also control what farmers get paid for crops and livestock, and the final price consumers eventually pay for food.

Many large food corporations are using their power to *expand* monocultures in crops and livestock production. As a result, individual farmers are subject to the demands of a few large food and biotech corporations who often make them sign contracts dictating the way their products must be grown or raised. For example, a food company can require farmers to use a proprietary food mix as animal feed, and the farmer may never know exactly what's in it. Or a seed company can prevent the farmer from saving their seeds from year to year, ending an age-old farming tradition. The contracts can undermine the farmer's expertise and may go against basic principles they've used for generations.

In order to support the high demand for our processed food system in the United States, many American farmers are now planting genetically modified crops and operating factory farms. The seeds, planting, and harvesting of our food crops are often controlled through patents and contracts—not the farmers' lessons learned through generations of sustainable farming. The living conditions, treatment, and feed of livestock and poultry are also controlled through contracts, not the farmers' experience from raising healthy animals in a sustainable way that produces a quality food product. Many farmers have suffered both emotional and financial turmoil in trying to deal with the pressures they feel from some in the food and biotech industries. Needless to say, all of these changes have undermined the critical role of the American farmer and many of the final food products we feed our children—and made it especially difficult for independent farms to survive.

Sadly, we've lost many American farmers during the past few decades, but their rich farming traditions live on through the perseverance of independent organic and sustainable farmers. Although industrialized agriculture still drives our food system, public awareness of these problems is building strong support for reforms.

Section 5: Food and Health

The doctor of the future will give no medicine, but will interest his patients in the care of the human frame, in diet, and in the cause and prevention of disease.
—Thomas Edison

Over the past few decades we have increased the use of food additives, rolled out more and more GMO products, and produced the vast majority of our meat and dairy in factory farms. With so many changes, is it any wonder that food could be at the root of many of our children's health problems?

DISCOVERING THE SOURCE (MARGARET)

As a young teen, my daughter Maggie experienced a chronic cough and was diagnosed with asthma. A doctor instructed her to never go anywhere without her inhaler. He prescribed it for daily use and although my husband and I were concerned about the long-term effects of this, we followed the doctor's orders. The following year Maggie began having severe stomach pains, and after several trips to the physician, she received no diagnosis. She was, however, encouraged to keep a food diary and record everything she was eating, noting when symptoms occurred. It didn't take Maggie long to notice that gluten (a protein found in wheat, barley, and rye) seemed to be causing the problem. We returned to the doctors and learned that Maggie was experiencing gluten sensitivity. Once all gluten was removed from her diet, not only did her stomach pains disappear, but all symptoms related to her chronic asthma as well.

The field of environmental medicine explores the interaction between people and their environment and how this interaction influences the development and progression of human disease. Environmental medicine is a specialty field of medicine practiced by licensed physicians. They examine many environmental factors our children are exposed to (including food) and the potential adverse effects these factors may be having on their health, well-being, or behaviors.

For centuries, dietary interventions have been used to treat a variety of health problems, but these days it's less commonly employed because other more convenient medical and pharmaceutical interventions are often available. It's very reassuring that environmental medicine and other holistic health practitioners *still* use food and diet as an integral part of their overall health assessment. They often routinely test for food allergies and food sensitivities in children with chronic health issues—even when no gastrointestinal (GI) symptoms are present— because food can have far-reaching effects on the human body well beyond the GI tract. These tests can provide clues and connections to various symptoms and health effects children experience from their diet.

Like many mothers, we both found food to be a contributing factor to our own children's chronic health problems. For example, when Joanne's son Colin removed sugary drinks from his diet as a teenager, his chronic migraine headaches improved. When Christine's daughter Kaleigh was taken off all processed food as a toddler, her eczema and asthma cleared up, and her thin brittle hair began to grow in thick and beautiful. All too often when suspect foods are identified and taken out of the diet, symptoms subside. Many scientific studies are supporting these findings as well. Below is just one example highlighting how food may play a role in children's chronic health problems. We found an interesting (albeit small) study conducted at Georgetown University School of Medicine and published in September 1994 edition of *Annuals of Allergy*. The "Did You Know?" below provides some background information.

Did You Know?

- Over 70 percent of American infants have been given at least one course of *antibiotics* by the age of six months.
- Many of these antibiotics are prescribed for *ear infections*.
- Over *half a million children* each year have tubes surgically placed in their ears because of chronic ear infections.

The Georgetown University School of Medicine study indicated that *food allergies* may be a key factor in many recurrent infections. Researchers discovered that 81 of the 104 children who participated in the recurrent ear infection study were allergic to various foods. Approximately one-third had an allergy to milk and another one-third was affected by wheat. Parents were instructed to keep their children *off* the offending food for four months. The result? Seventy of the children improved with significant clearing of the ears. Parents were then instructed to put the offending foods *back* into the diet of their children. The result? Within four months, 66 of the children had clogged ears again. Researchers

for the study attributed the excess mucus production and swelling of
the middle ear tube (which resulted in recurrent ear infections) to food
allergies.

Although an extremely small study, it shows a powerful cause and effect with
dietary interventions when identified food allergies or sensitivities play a role. It
clearly shows us that often times we can get to the root of the problem and offer
an alternative approach to merely treating symptoms of an illness. How many
of our children are unknowingly being affected by food choices? How many
of our children possibly underwent surgical ear tube placement unnecessarily?
Environmental medicine is often used in conjunction with traditional medical
practices to provide more balanced and comprehensive care. See the Resource
Guide in Part 3 or at www.behindcloseddoorsthebook.com for more information
on environmental medicine and how to locate a doctor practicing it in your area.

A HEALING PARTNERSHIP (CHRISTINE)

When Kaleigh was twenty months old, we were vacationing with my
in-laws at the beach in Ocean City, New Jersey. My husband John was
in the ocean with Kaleigh when she suddenly began to develop hives.
I saw John's panicked face as he was walking toward me, and I jumped
into action, questioning all of our relatives and my children to see if
Kaleigh had eaten or drunk something off-limits. She hadn't and I then
realized she was most likely reacting to something in the ocean. That
night I cried myself to sleep, thinking what my child's life would be like
if she could have an allergic reaction to a natural body of water. Both my
husband and I felt powerless, but knew we had to do something.

The next morning, I was determined to find answers. I began doing
more research and learned about digestive enzymes and how important
they are for our digestive system, which I already suspected was the root
cause of Kaleigh's health issues. This led me to a book called The Food
Allergy Cure by Dr. Ellen Cutler, MD, and to an alternative modality
called Namudripad's Allergy Elimination Techniques (NAET), a
program of desensitization that can help individuals with food allergies.
I began looking for a NAET practitioner in my area. The next day I was

having lunch with Joanne's sister. We began discussing our children's health, and she told me about a local practitioner she used for her own daughter, who practiced this technique.

I can still remember the day I walked into this doctor's office with my toddler in my arms. The woman's warm smile and caring presence put me at ease right away. She reviewed Kaleigh's medical history and diagnoses and began to develop an individualized protocol.

"We are going to do this together," she said. "I'm going to give you the tools, but you're going to use them to help your daughter get better."

I felt such relief and so much hope welling up in my heart. I was grateful we'd reached a turning point in restoring Kaleigh.

Over the next two years, I drove an hour every other week to this holistic practitioner. It took time for Kaleigh's autoimmune system to heal, but we were making progress. During this period, we utilized the help of many health practitioners both traditional and holistic. I certainly took advantage of all that conventional medicine had to offer. But it was not enough. It wasn't until I started implementing an integrative protocol of nutrition, digestive enzymes, vitamins, minerals, NAET, and detoxification that we began to see steady improvements. Kaleigh's eczema began to disappear and her face cleared up—no more bleeding! Her hair began to change from dry and stringy to thick, curly, and beautiful. We also didn't need the nebulizer for her asthma nearly as often now.

When Kaleigh had a new biomedical analysis, many of the heavy metals and toxins present within her a year earlier were significantly lower. I felt so empowered and grateful to have met this doctor, but every time I thanked her, she just smiled and said, "We are doing it together."

My baby girl was healing right in front of my eyes.

Although most of us aren't fully aware of all that's been playing out behind closed doors in the food industry, some of us have started to learn more through important documentaries like *Food Inc.* and important books like *The Unhealthy*

Truth, and *Altered Genes, Twisted Truth.* Yet these alarming reports rarely make front-page news. We need to understand just how out of balance some of our newer food practices have become and the detrimental toll they have taken on our children's health. Only by facing the truth of what is happening can we become empowered to change it. It will take the voice of each and everyone one of us standing together as mothers and parents to let the entire food industry know that reforms are needed and change must come.

Chapter 6

THE PHARMACEUTICAL INDUSTRY

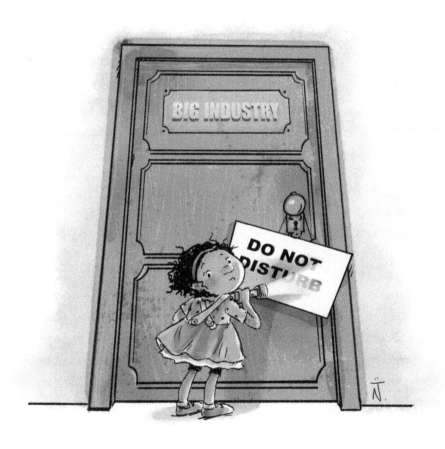

Truth never damages a cause that is just.
—Mohandas Gandhi

I f we're going to evaluate children's health and well-being, we need to address the topic of pharmaceuticals. Pharmaceuticals were first developed in the twentieth century and have provided us with breakthrough medical advancements that not only save lives but also greatly improve the quality of life for many. It goes without saying that many people rely on lifesaving pharmaceutical treatments. However, the pharmaceutical industry has ballooned over the last one hundred years, and, as moms, we can't help but ask has it grown out of balance? Are some treatments that started out in an effort to help now causing some harm along the way? The topic of pharmaceutical treatment is vast, so in this chapter, we have chosen to focus on the two areas that have undergone some of the biggest changes over the past few decades, potentially impacting the largest number of children: vaccines and mental health treatments.

Section 1: Childhood Vaccine Practices

The subject of childhood vaccines has been surrounded by much debate and controversy. As authors, our own individual views on vaccines even split us a little. When discussing vaccines, we feel it is important to remember that we all have our children's best interest at heart. Whether a parent decides to vaccinate, selectively vaccinate, or not vaccinate at all, each one feels that their choice best protects the health and well-being of their child.

During a measles outbreak in early 2015, we got a chance to sit down with Bridget, a mother of two young daughters who's also a family nurse practitioner and a college nursing instructor. She was upset by the strong rift among parents and even between parents and healthcare providers over the subject of vaccines. When she spoke so simply and honestly about the issue, we knew her thoughts needed to be shared.

WHERE'S THE COMMON SENSE? (BRIDGET)

As parents we care deeply about what goes into our children's bodies. We try to give them fresh food without preservatives, pesticides, and GMOs. We lather on natural mineral-based sunscreen and listen to our healthcare provider's advice about the harms of the inappropriate use of antibiotics or the overuse of acetaminophen and ibuprofen. We breastfeed our babies and as nursing mothers we watch what we eat and what we put on and into our own bodies. As parents, we diligently check every label of food we give our child and every soap and lotion we use on them. So, naturally as parents we can't help but to check the label of vaccines that are injected into our children. It's part of a habit of care.

When parents look at a vaccine label and see these ingredients—formaldehyde, egg protein, monosodium glutamate, thimerosal, aluminum, antibiotics, yeast protein, monkey kidney tissue, and the list goes on—it defies common sense. Is it any wonder parents are in a quandary?

Vaccinations have played an important role in protecting our children from infectious disease and hold a significant place in public health practices, especially for many at-risk populations. However, our U.S. childhood vaccination program has gone through many changes over the past few decades. One of the biggest is that we've more than *tripled* the number of required vaccinations for children—during that same time period children's health outcomes have worsened in many areas. Some may find it uncomfortable to question vaccines in any way, but we believe there is nothing wrong with exploring any of our practices, public health ones included. This does not make us antivaccine, any more than it makes us anticar when questioning vehicle safety. Questioning is how most reform begins. We're not taking a stand for or against vaccinations. We're merely looking at important vaccine facts that lack transparency so that we can shed light on areas in need of reform and become more informed parents making more informed decisions.

One reason we feel that this topic is so emotionally charged is because as mothers and parents we'd never place our child in harm's way. Yet we're told by those on both sides of the vaccine issue that our child can be harmed by our choice to vaccinate or not to vaccinate. Where does this leave us? The fact remains that there are known risks on both sides of the issue, which puts us in a daunting position as protectors of our children.

Just as food is a big business, so too are pharmaceuticals, and we're consumers of both. Pharmaceutical companies undoubtedly have large promotional budgets and due to the very nature of the business, they also have close ties with federal agencies charged with vaccine oversight. Because both have a vested interest in promoting vaccines, it often results in public relations that focus on the benefits of vaccinations to a far greater extent than addressing the potential risks. We have the right to balanced information so that we can make an informed decision in the best interest of our children. Let's start by examining what our childhood vaccine program looked like thirty years ago and what it looks like today.

U.S. Vaccine Schedule
from Birth to Kindergarten
1983 vs. TODAY

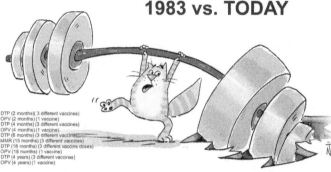

Hep B (birth) (1 vaccine)
Hep B (1 month) (1 vaccine)
DTap (2 months) (3 different vaccines)
Hib (2 months) (1 vaccine)
IPV (2 months) (1 vaccine)
PCV (2 months) (1 vaccine)
Rotavirus (2 months) (1 vaccine)
DTap (4 months) (3 different vaccines)
Hib (4 months) (1 vaccine)
IPV (4 months) (1 vaccine)
PCV (4 months) (1 vaccine)
Rotavirus (4 months) (1 vaccine)
Hep B (6 months) (1 vaccine)
DTap (6 months) (3 different vaccines)
Hib (6 months) (1 vaccine)
IPV (6 months) (1 vaccine)
PCV (6 months) (1 vaccine)
Rotavirus (6 months) (1 vaccine)
Influenza (6 months) (1 vaccine)
Influenza (7 months) (1 vaccine)
Hib (12 months) (1 vaccine)
MMR (12 months) (3 different vaccines)
Varicella (12 months) (1 vaccine)
PCV (12 months) (1 vaccine)
HepA(12 months) (1 vaccine)
DTaP(15 months) (3 different vaccines)
HepA(18 months) (1 vaccine)
Influenza (18 months) (1 vaccine)
PPSV only if high risk (2 years - 1 vaccine)
MCV only if high risk (2 years - 1 vaccine)
Influenza (2 ½ years) (1 vaccine)
Influenza (3 ½ years) (1 vaccine)
MMR (4 years) (3 different vaccines)
DTaP (4 years) (3 different vaccines)
Varicella (4 years) (1 vaccine)
IPV (4 years) (1 vaccine)
Influenza (4 ½ years) (1 vaccine)

DTP (2 months)(3 different vaccines)
OPV (2 months) (1 vaccine)
DTP (4 months) (3 different vaccines)
OPV (4 months) (1 vaccine)
DTP (6 months) (3 different vaccines)
MMR (15 months) (3 different vaccines)
DTP (18 months) (3 different vaccine doses)
OPV (18 months) (1 vaccine)
DTP (4 years) (3 different vaccines)
OPV (4 years) (1 vaccine)

1983
10 shots
(22 different vaccine doses)

2015
35-37 shots
(49-51 different vaccine doses)

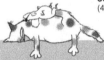

All before Our Child's First Day of Kindergarten

▷ Are we **over** vaccinating?

▷ **26** vaccine doses are now administered before our child's **1st birthday.**

▷ **50** vaccine doses may now be administered before our child's **1st day** of **kindergarten.**

▷ Is the **increased** use of vaccines burdening the **immune system** of developing children?

▷ Is the **increased** use of vaccines contributing to **chronic health problems** in our children?

Sources: Data for both the 1983 and 2015 Childhood Immunization Schedule were from the Centers for Disease Control and Prevention (CDC). [*Authors' notes: Kindergarten is defined as age 5. Prior to 1995, vaccine schedules were only published periodically.*]

MORE THAN ENOUGH (CHRISTINE)

In the summer of 2014, my family and I took a trip to Ireland. On the way, we stopped in London to visit Kaleigh's friend Rachel and her family for a few days. Our friends had just moved back to London, their native home, after living in the States for the past decade or so. During our visit, Rachel's mom and I began discussing vaccines. I'd brought up the subject, as I was curious to hear about the vaccine protocol in the UK.

Rachel's mom has a really good sense of humor. Despite the seriousness of this subject, she couldn't help but chuckle when she recounted her experience at the doctor's office after giving the physician and his nurse her daughter's vaccine records.

"They stared at it wide-eyed," she recounted, "and with funny looks on their faces. When I asked if there was anything wrong, or if Rachel was behind on something, the nurse replied a bit sarcastically, 'No, we think your daughter has had enough vaccines to last her a lifetime, and then some.'"

Is Our Vaccine Schedule Growing Out of Balance?

When looking at the changes in the U.S. childhood vaccination schedule, one can't help but wonder if we are we overusing the vaccine technology we have been afforded. Over the past few decades, we've learned some important lessons from possible overuse and abuse in medicine. Antibiotics and C-Section births are two perfect examples. We took an abundance of antibiotics, one of medicine's greatest achievements, and have slowly destroyed their power through widespread overuse in both humans and animals—resulting in the very serious public health problem of antibiotic resistance in humans.

Another practice many now feel that we began to use for convenience rather than necessity is C-section births. It can be lifesaving technology, but also puts both mothers and infants at higher risk for birth complications. Since we began routinely using C-section births, our maternal death rate has also increased. The over use of C-sections has been identified as one possible contributing factor, and efforts to ensure they're only being used when medically necessary have now been implemented. Similarly, we need to ensure that our childhood vaccination programs—designed to save lives—are not growing out of balance and causing unintended harm along the way.

In the same way that C-section deliveries may not be warranted for every birth, a growing number of parents believe that certain infant vaccinations currently on the recommended schedule may not be warranted for every child in America. Vaccine availability shouldn't automatically equate to mandated use in every child. An example of just one vaccine many parents question is the immunization for hepatitis B recommended at birth for all U.S infants. This particular vaccine really only *needs* to be administered to infants born to mothers who test positive for the disease, because hepatitis B is most commonly transmitted by sex and intravenous (I.V.) drug use. This is one vaccine a newborn's body may be able to do without at least until they are much older—as is the practice in many other countries, with some countries not requiring it at all. Yet, here in the United States, we administer the hepatitis B vaccine when our babies are only hours old. The most controversial aspect of the hepatitis B vaccine is that given at birth it will deliver the highest dose per pound of the vaccine ingredient (and brain toxin) aluminum to our newborns, and potentially unnecessarily. Where is the common sense in this practice?

Let us remind you that U.S. vaccine protocols are *not* the norm. We are the *most* vaccinated country in the world. Yet our children's health statistics are worsening in many areas with more children suffering from chronic illnesses than ever before. We're questioning if the increased number of vaccines our children receive plays any role at all in these statistical realities. In the United States we have twenty-six recommended vaccine doses for infants in the first twelve months of life. That's *double* what's currently required for infants in many other countries. Maybe we need to take a step back and look at the health outcomes our current childhood vaccination schedule is producing and ask ourselves if this practice is in balance and serving our children well. For starters, is it really necessary to expose an infant to so many different vaccines on the same day? Currently, nine different vaccine doses are recommended to be administered to an infant at the six-month visit. Is the timing and dosing for all these simultaneous vaccines tested and safe? Is every single vaccination on the current schedule really necessary to recommend for every single child in America? What are the long-term effects of the increased vaccination schedule on a developing immune system?

A recent independent study looked specifically at many of these same questions surrounding the safety of the current childhood schedule and possible long-term health outcomes. The study report noted that although the existing evidence is reassuring, safety questions still remain largely unanswered because not enough studies in this area have been conducted.

Did You Know?

 The National Vaccine Program Office (NVPO) of the U.S. Department of Health and Human Services (HHS) asked the Institute of Medicine (IOM) to convene a committee of experts to look at the *scientific evidence* supporting the recommended childhood vaccination schedule. In 2013, the IOM issued their report based on a twelve-month evaluation. In this report, *The Childhood Immunization Schedule and Safety: Stakeholders Concerns, Scientific Evidence and Future Studies*, the committee found no significant scientific evidence to imply that the recommended immunization schedule is *not* safe. However, the IOM committee repeatedly noted there was a *lack* of quality scientific studies to *support* the *safety* of the recommended timing and doses of vaccinations on the schedule for children in the 0–6 age group. For example, studies designed to examine the long-term effects of the cumulative number of vaccines and many other aspects of the immunization schedule have not been conducted. The report also noted that there were large knowledge gaps concerning children with the potential for increased susceptibility to vaccine reactions and injuries. Many significant considerations for future research examining the different components of the vaccine schedule and its relationship to adverse events and long-term health outcomes were proposed.

Just as it is important to know where your children's food comes from it is also important to know where your children's vaccines come from. As young mothers, we certainly knew about the benefits of childhood immunizations. However, we were much less informed about the associated risks. The way vaccines are manufactured and the ingredients vaccines contain shed light on these risks. In the next section we explore vaccine ingredients to see if they could be impacting our children's health in any way. We have also provided some practical tools that may offer concerned parents greater confidence when vaccinating. You can find additional resources and references on many of the vaccine topics in the Resource Guide in Part 3 or at www. behindcloseddoorsthebook.com.

Section 2: What Goes into Our Children's Vaccines?

> *If you can't convince them, confuse them.*
> —Harry Truman

Vaccinations are important forms of prophylactic medication because they can help prevent disease. However, it's important to know that vaccines are not drugs. They are *biologics* and carry risks much different from conventional drugs due to the ingredients they contain and the way they're made. Biologics are manufactured in a living system. The process often requires growing viruses used in the vaccines in human tissue or animal tissue (such as a monkey kidney), resulting in the risk of possible cross-contamination. For example, if the human or animal tissue was infected with a disease, it could contaminate the final vaccination a child receives. Naturally, the FDA requires that many precautions be taken to prevent this, but cross-contamination with animal viruses has happened in the past.

Many different ingredients are used in developing a vaccination and each ingredient serves an important purpose. Ingredients differ for specific vaccines, but can also differ for the *same* vaccine type, depending on the manufacturer (e.g., Merck or Eli Lilly). It's empowering to know that we sometimes have vaccine *brand choices*, just as we have brand choices at the food store. While there are many different vaccine ingredients, we'll closely examine only two of them, the preservative thimerosal (*still used* in some vaccines) and the adjuvant, aluminum. These aren't contained in all vaccines, so we encourage you to learn more about the ingredients contained in each individual vaccine your child receives and the potential health effects. For a sample list of what a vaccine may contain and where to find the most reliable information on vaccine ingredients (manufacturer's product inserts), see the Resource Guide in Part 3 or at www.behindcloseddoorsthebook.com.

Thimerosal: Going, Going, but Still Not Gone!

Preservatives are used to prevent microbial contamination of the vaccine and are required for vaccines contained in multidose vials (they contain enough vaccine to use for several shots and are often more cost-effective than single-dose vaccines). Thimerosal is one example of a preservative used in some vaccines. Thimerosal is about 50 percent mercury (ethylmercury) by weight. Mercury is one of the most toxic elements on earth and even in low doses can cause nervous system and brain damage, an effect that has been well documented in medical literature.

The controversy over the use of thimerosal in vaccines began when FDA legislation was introduced in 1997, requiring a closer look at levels of heavy metals used in food and medicine. This legislation forced vaccine policymakers to do the math on *cumulative levels* of exposure through our children's ever-growing vaccination schedule, which no one had ever bothered to do. As a result, The House Committee on Government Reform initiated an investigation into the potential dangers of mercury exposure through the expanding vaccination schedule. In July of 2000, it was estimated that about 8,000 children a day were being exposed to mercury in excess of federal guidelines through these schedules. Needless to say, this was not what those in charge of vaccine oversight wanted to hear, and some families feel they have suffered tragic health consequences as a result.

The FDA and EPA have since handed down a directive to the pharmaceutical industry that led to the removal of thimerosal from *most* vaccinations. However, thimerosal *remains* in a few vaccines, including some brands of the flu, tetanus, and meningitis vaccines at levels exceeding federal guidelines, and also remains in trace amounts in other vaccines. Infants receiving a thimerosal-containing influenza vaccine are dosed at six months with 12.5 micrograms (mcg) of ethyl mercury and at seven months with an additional 12.5 mcg. A fifteen-pound baby receiving a thimerosal-containing vaccine would far exceed the EPA reference dose for safety (set at *0.1 micrograms* per kilogram of body weight per day). More than twenty years ago, Russia *banned* thimerosal from use in childhood vaccinations due to safety concerns, and Japan, Austria, Great Britain, and all of the Scandinavian countries have since done the same. The entire European Union has also phased it out.

Yet today some flu vaccinations offered to American children contain 25 micrograms of thimerosal, exposing them to a dose of ethylmercury exceeding the government recommended safety threshold. Why are flu shots containing thimerosal even *offered* to children or pregnant women when thimerosal-free alternatives are available? Thankfully, California and Iowa have banned the use of thimerosal in vaccines for pregnant women, and children under the age of three. Over thirty states are working towards similar bans. The good news is that today you can completely avoid thimerosal by understanding your brand choices. More details are provided in our vaccine practical tools found in Section 4.

*[Authors' note: Because there are no safety guidelines set for ethylmercury (the metabolite of thimerosal), the FDA considers ethyl and methylmercury as equivalent in its risk evaluation. The EPA reference dose limit for methylmercury is **0.1 micrograms (mcg) per kilogram of body weight per day**. A fifteen-pound baby is equivalent to weighing about seven kilograms, exceeding the limit many times over.]*

Aluminum: Trading One Toxic Ingredient for Another

Aluminum is used as an adjuvant in some childhood vaccines. An adjuvant allows the vaccine to produce a stronger antibody response and to be more effective. When thimerosal was phased out from *most* childhood vaccinations, new vaccines containing high doses of aluminum were phased in. Aluminum is highly toxic to our children's brains, even in small amounts, and like thimerosal can pose a threat for neurological and immune-related problems. Is this why we didn't see a big decrease in neurodevelopmental problems in our infants and children once thimerosal began to be removed? Have we merely traded one toxic substance for another?

When we raise potential concerns about aluminum with our healthcare providers, we're often told about all the other ways children are exposed to aluminum in our water, air, and food. Yet there's a big difference between these other exposures and what is *injected* into the bodies of our children through vaccines. Injected aluminum is far more dangerous because 100 percent of it is expected to be absorbed from the muscle into the bloodstream. When aluminum is taken into the body in food, the gastrointestinal tract acts as a significant barrier to absorption into the blood. Additionally, injected aluminum remains in the body for much longer periods of time, while aluminum from diet is excreted rapidly. Because of the known health hazards of *injectable* aluminum, the FDA now requires a warning label on all forms of injectable aluminum medicine products, which says, "This product contains aluminum that may be toxic."

Intravenous hydration solutions (dextrose solutions) contain aluminum and carry this warning due to potential aluminum toxicity. Intravenous nutritional supplement solutions (TPN) that contain aluminum carry the same label. Yet vaccines containing aluminum *aren't* required to carry the warning label or meet these limits. Why not?

Warning labels for TPN also limit the amount of aluminum the product can contain to 25 mcg/per liter. The warning also references safe limits set for the amount of injected aluminum a person can receive depending on their body weight. Once again, vaccines do not follow these FDA guidelines. Why not?

When we follow the current childhood vaccination schedule, it's possible to far exceed the stringent safety guidelines set by the FDA for other forms of injectable medicine containing aluminum. For example, if the hepatitis B vaccination, given at birth and containing 250 mcg of aluminum, was administered to an 8-pound infant, it would *exceed by ten times* other FDA safety regulations set for injectable aluminum medicine. Where is the common sense in this?

According to the American Society for Parental and Enteral Nutrition, studies suggest that aluminum in *injectable form* can build up in the bloodstream, bone, and brain to toxic levels in premature infants. We don't know if this is true for healthy full-term infants because aluminum as a vaccine adjuvant—at levels our children have been exposed to—has never undergone any human safety testing to see how it's absorbed into their bloodstream or may affect their bodies. Concerns about the safety of aluminum in vaccines have been raised repeatedly in medical literature. The following is just one excerpt from a 2011 peer-reviewed journal article in *Current Medicinal Chemistry*:

> Experimental research clearly shows that aluminum adjuvants have a potential to induce serious immunological disorders in humans. In particular, aluminum in adjuvant form carries a risk for autoimmunity, long-term brain inflammation and associated neurological complications and may thus have profound and widespread adverse health consequences.

One in six U.S. children currently has developmental difficulties, from a subtle learning disability to behavioral or emotional disorders. We're in the midst of an autism epidemic and autoimmune disorders such as asthma, allergies, juvenile diabetes, arthritis, and more are on the rise. Are we witnessing the potential long-term health consequences noted in this peer-reviewed medical journal? There appears to be a growing number of children who are more susceptible to toxins than others, including those toxins found in vaccine adjuvants, like aluminum. Should we factor an infant or child's body weight into the safety equation of vaccines containing aluminum as other federal guidelines do? Can we develop ways to screen children for vaccine sensitivities prior to immunizations? Does our one-size-fits-all schedule account for the unique needs of every child? Efforts and continued conversations in these areas can improve vaccine safety and possibly improve health outcomes in our children.

To summarize, the FDA has determined that a *single dose* of vaccine is permitted to contain more than *ten times* the limit set for other injectable aluminum products. If we follow the current vaccination schedule, with several visits during the first year of life, our infants may receive *multiple* shots in one day that each contain aluminum. What will the cumulative effect be at the time of the shots? Who does this guideline serve?

*[Authors' notes: No aluminum clinical studies have been conducted in healthy infants and children to **prove** either safety or harm. The FDA suggests limiting injected aluminum content to 25 mcg/per liter. Recommended safety limits of 5 mcg of aluminum per every kg of weight are also made for vulnerable populations. As a reference point, an 8-pound infant is 3.6 kg (rounded up is 4 kg) equating to a 20 mcg limit. The hepatitis B vaccine given at birth contains 250 mcg. See the Resource Guide for an Aluminum Supplement containing additional details including a list of vaccines that contain aluminum and the amounts they contain.]*

The Combined and Cumulative Effect: Are Vaccine Ingredients Adding Up?

It is important to state once again that vaccinations can help prevent the spread of infectious disease, and both the FDA and the Centers for Disease Control and Prevention (CDC) state that the benefits of vaccines outweigh the risks. However, risks do exist and although the current research is reassuring, many questions regarding the safety of individual vaccine ingredients, the current childhood schedule, and potential long-term health outcomes are still unanswered.

Below is an excerpt from a 2012 article published in *Lupus*, an international, peer-reviewed journal that raises valid concerns about vaccine ingredients our children are exposed to and best describes the potential dangers and health effects less commonly known to parents.

> Immune challenges during early development, including those vaccine-induced, can lead to permanent detrimental alterations of the brain and immune function. Experimental evidence also shows that simultaneous administration of as little as two to three immune adjuvants can overcome genetic resistance to autoimmunity. In some developed countries, by the time children are 4 to 6 years old, they will have received a total of 126 antigenic compounds along with high amounts of aluminum (Al) adjuvants through routine vaccinations. According to the US Food and Drug Administration, safety assessments for vaccines have often not included appropriate toxicity studies because vaccines have

not been viewed as inherently toxic. Taken together, these observations raise plausible concerns about the overall safety of current childhood vaccination program.

Remember that the number of shots required of U.S. children has tripled over the past few decades—so the amount of vaccine ingredients infants and children are being subjected to has also increased substantially. Once again, it all adds up. We need to continue our conversations about this important topic until well-designed, independent safety studies are conducted and replicated ensuring that our children's ever-growing vaccine schedule is safe. Some practical tools you can easily implement to address concerns about vaccine ingredients appear at the end of Section 4.

RED FLAG (CHRISTINE)

My first three children did not appear to have any reactions to their childhood vaccines. However, Kaleigh was a different story. As my youngest child, the immunization schedule she followed was more intense than the one we followed for her siblings. I believe Kaleigh experienced a serious autoimmune reaction following her nine-month shots. Due to an array of chronic illnesses that immediately followed, I refused to follow the rigor of the recommended schedule for my children and began to do my own vaccine research. Several years later, I was at a sick visit with one of my children when the topic of "catching up" was raised. I immediately began to question the presence of specific vaccine ingredients I was concerned about for Kaleigh, who has proven to be highly sensitive to chemicals and other toxins. Before I could finish my first sentence, my doctor's hand went up to stop me from speaking any further.

"I don't know where you got that information from," she said, "but the only website you are to view is the CDC website."

I was shocked that my valid concerns about authentic vaccine ingredients didn't warrant a conversation. I was also angry that my ability to access valid health information was questioned and under censorship. The situation escalated and I was politely asked to leave the practice because I refused to follow the recommended vaccine schedule for my children. I left the practice and quickly found a wonderful family practice willing to engage in dialogue about my vaccine concerns and respected my right as a parent to make informed health decisions for my children. Any healthcare provider not willing to engage in dialogue about the health concerns you have regarding your children should be a red flag that it's time to find a new provider.

Section 3: Conflicts of Interest in Vaccines

If the people cannot trust their government to do the job for which it exists— to protect them and to promote their common welfare—all else is lost.
—President Obama

On February 8, 2005, the *Los Angeles Times* reported that a major cover-up took place regarding children's vaccine safety. In 1991, a researcher at a major pharmaceutical company discovered that the cumulative amount of mercury in vaccines given to infants by six months of age was about *87 times* the safety limits set by the FDA. According to the article, the researcher immediately informed those in charge of what he discovered via internal documents. However, no corrective action was immediately taken to protect those in danger. Instead, this information was kept behind closed doors and not revealed to the public until years later. It's unfathomable for most mothers to comprehend that those in the field of medicine were aware that possible neurological harm was occurring to our nation's infants while they sat silently protecting their public image and economic bottom line.

FAILURE AT THE TOP (JOANNE)

I never wrestled more with my background in public health than when confronting past reports about cover-ups regarding vaccines. As a medical writer working in the pharmaceutical industry, I had a difficult time digesting what I had uncovered, making this particular chapter especially difficult to write. It was disheartening to learn that those at the top, in places of power, were aware of potential safety issues, conflicts of interest, or other potential problems that could jeopardize consumers and did nothing about it. All the while, so many like myself, who work day in and day out in various aspects of pharmaceutical development are held to much higher standards of operation, where consumer safety is first and foremost in every procedure and policy we must follow.

Did You Know?

 In 1995 the CDC Foundation, which was created by Congress, began to accept "gifts" on behalf of the CDC. The *BMJ* (formerly the *British Medical Journal*), an international peer-reviewed medical journal, called out the conflicts of interest this foundation has promoted within the agency in a 2015 article: "Despite the agency's disclaimer, the CDC does receive millions of dollars in industry gifts and funding, both directly and indirectly, and several recent CDC actions and recommendations have raised questions about the science it cites, the clinical guidelines it promotes, and the money it is taking."

FDA and CDC Vaccine Advisory Committees

Currently, the same federal agencies that conduct vaccine safety research are also charged with developing and patenting vaccines, regulating their use, and making policy for vaccine promotions and distribution. During the past few decades, there's been an increased focus of concern surrounding the pharmaceutical industry's influence on medicine. As the U.S.-recommended childhood vaccine schedule continued to expand over the past thirty years, the FDA and CDC, who are both involved in vaccine oversight, also came under scrutiny for conflict-of-interest violations. Conflicts of interest *do not* always result in unethical practices, but they certainly can place a cloud of doubt over an entire system.

Pharmaceutical companies who manufacture vaccines have financial ties to the FDA and the CDC in a variety of ways. Due to these financial relationships, concerns became so serious about potential conflicts of interest that Congressional hearings were eventually held. Most notable was one in 2000 that focused on those who participate on vaccine advisory committees for both the FDA (Vaccine and Related Biological Products Advisory Committee) and the CDC (Advisory Committee on Immunization Practices). In 2003, another Congressional Report and hearing also exposed additional conflicts of interest in vaccine policymaking. The decisions of these committees have impacted every child in America. The FDA committee noted above approves and licenses pharmaceutical companies' vaccines, and the CDC committee above makes recommendations on which vaccines should be included on the childhood vaccine schedule. Here are some examples of what the 2000 hearing before the Committee of Government Reform exposed about these committees:

- Members of the FDA and CDC vaccine advisory committees making decisions regarding the health and well-being of our children owned stock in drug companies that make the vaccines. (*They could personally profit from the decisions their committee made to approve a vaccine or place a vaccine on the U.S. schedule.*)
- Individuals on both vaccine advisory committees *owned patents* for vaccines that were under consideration or affected by the decisions of the committee. (*They owned or partially owned the rights to the vaccine—so they could undoubtedly profit from the decisions the committee made to approve **their own vaccine** or place **their own vaccine** on the U.S. schedule.*)
- Although conflict-of-interest rules exist to protect the integrity of the process, the CDC routinely grants conflict-of-interest *waivers* that are valid for a year at a time to every member of their advisory committee. Members who have a financial stake in pending decisions are allowed full participation in the discussions leading up to a vote. (*So those that stood to profit from the committee's decisions were allowed to influence other committee members.*)
- The FDA grants conflict-of-interest waivers to members of their vaccine advisory committee who have financial conflicts of interest, permitting them to still be a voting member. (*They could vote with a waiver if they*

had financial conflicts—but waivers were not granted if the vaccine was their own.)

In 2003, another report exposing additional CDC and FDA vaccine conflicts of interest was released. This time is was concerning the dangers of mercury exposure through vaccinations. Here are just a few of the findings in the 2003 Congressional Report *Mercury in Medicine, Taking Unnecessary Risks*:

- The FDA never required the pharmaceutical industry to conduct extensive safety studies on thimerosal or ethylmercury even though the possible risk for harm from either low-dose chronic exposure or high-level one-time exposure to thimerosal was not "theoretical," but very real and documented in the medical literature.
- The CDC in general and the National Immunization Program in particular are *conflicted* in their duties to monitor the safety of vaccines, while also charged with the responsibility of purchasing vaccines for resale as well as promoting increased immunization rates.
- The CDC's ability to look fairly at emerging theories and clinical data related to adverse reactions from vaccinations was called into question.

While improvements have been implemented since these hearings, conflicts of interest *still* exist, and our vaccine advisory committees are still permitted to make some conflict-of-interest exceptions using waiver loopholes. In a more recent 2009 report, issued by the inspector general of the Department of Health and Human Services and titled *CDC's Ethics Program for Special Government Employees on Federal Advisory Committees,* the CDC was found to have inadequately screened medical experts for financial conflicts when they were hired to advise the CDC on vaccine safety in 2007. Sixty-four percent of these special employees had potential conflicts of interest that were either never identified or left unresolved by the Centers and 3 percent voted on particular matters that an ethics officer had prohibited them from participating in. Most of these experts served on vaccine advisory panels.

Late in 2009, the Director of the CDC resigned her post at the CDC to head the vaccine division at Merck, the world's largest vaccine manufacturer. This is a classic example of what has been referred to as a "revolving door" between those working in government agencies charged with oversight and the pharmaceutical industry. Many argue that this lack of separation between the regulators and the regulated compromises both scientific integrity and government accountability. We need reforms that allow us to have faith in the system and confidence that the safety of our children will come before any underlying political agenda or financial interest.

Did You Know?

 The *oral polio vaccine* was taken off the market in the early 2000s because the vaccine was actually *causing polio* in some of the children that were vaccinated. According to the CDC, the live-virus polio *vaccine* had become the dominant *cause* of polio in the United States and was responsible for about eight to nine cases yearly. The oral polio vaccine was removed from the immunization schedule and replaced with the injected, *inactivated* form of the vaccine so that children are *no long*er at risk for contracting polio from the vaccination. This is an excellent example of a vaccine reform.

GETTING THE BRUSH OFF (JOANNE)

While at the hairdresser's one day, a stylist shared with me how her infant son, who'd never had any neurological issues, had a full-blown seizure a few hours after receiving several scheduled immunizations. She went directly to the emergency room and followed up with her pediatrician. The pediatrician told her that the seizure was purely coincidental and not at all related to her son's vaccinations.

As a pharmaceutical medical writer, I often write patient narratives. These regulatory documents include every serious and sometimes nonserious adverse event that patients experience while

taking a newly developed drug, as part of a clinical trial. This information is part of a clinical study report that the FDA reviews before making decisions about a drug's approval. It disturbs me to hear mothers' stories about how their child's reported symptoms following vaccines were brushed aside. Adverse reactions are real, and I can tell you firsthand that the FDA and pharmaceutical companies take them very seriously.

I can't help but wonder if doctors are receiving balanced vaccine information. How can a healthcare provider be unaware of the potential for neurological problems following vaccines? Some of the reactions mothers have reported to me as being dismissed by healthcare providers are listed as potential reactions in the prescribing package inserts that accompany the vaccines and are well documented in medical literature. What additional harm are children being subjected to when they return for a second or third dose of the same vaccine after the first signs of a potential serious reaction were brushed off?

You can never overestimate the importance of transparency. One time Patrick and I were at University of Pennsylvania Hospital seeing an Ear, Nose, and Throat doctor. He knew Patrick's history and informed me that his most recent audiology test showed a continual decline in hearing—par for the course for the cancer treatment regimen he received.

"Radiation is the gift that keeps on giving," he said in a matter-of-fact way.

"Yes, I know that well," I replied.

He said I was one of the few "informed" parents of young adult brain tumor survivors and added, "I'm always amazed that families come into my office completely surprised that radiation to the brain could have such a profound effect on hearing so long after radiation has taken place. It's well documented in the medical journals. The oncology radiologists are the ones informing 'us' of the risks. So why do so many parents seem so surprised when it happens?"

Information is power.

Did You Know?

Direct-to-consumer pharmaceutical advertising (DTCPA) is an effort made by a pharmaceutical company to promote their prescription products directly to *patients*, most often through popular media such as TV, radio, and magazines. Most other countries don't allow this. Yet, here in the United States, this type of advertising has grown rapidly during the past several decades and is now the most common type of health communication that the public encounters. The United States and New Zealand are the only two countries in the world that permit DTCPA with product claims.

Section 4: Vaccine Facts Lack Transparency

Help me to disagree without blame, to share without criticism, and to debate without demonizing anyone.
—Marianne Williamson, *A Year of Miracles*

We feel that many important vaccine facts are not as transparent as they should be, undermining our rights as parents. So in this section we share some information to help you make more informed vaccine decisions.

Vaccine Safety and Efficacy

According to the FDA, vaccines undergo a thorough review of laboratory and clinical data to ensure the vaccine's relative safety, efficacy, purity, and potency before being marketed to the public. The FDA believes that the benefits of vaccinations outweigh the risk of serious health effects. With that being said, please be informed that some vaccine risks do exist.

Effectiveness: Each vaccine's rate of effectiveness will vary, but the CDC reports that *most* fall between 85 and –95 percent when all shots in a series are completed. However, some individual vaccine's effectiveness rates are quite low. For example, according to the CDC, the 2014–15 flu shot only had a 23 percent rate of effectiveness in reducing the risk of the influenza virus. In general, that means it was expected to *work* in 23 percent of those who received it. It also meant that it was *not expected to work* in 77 percent of those who received it. Getting a vaccination does not guarantee that it will provide immunity to the infectious disease it was designed to combat. Your child can be vaccinated for a particular disease and still contract that disease. We need to remain vigilant in watching for signs and symptoms of infectious disease during any outbreak—even when our child is fully vaccinated. A vaccine's rate of effectiveness will not appear on Vaccine Information Sheets (VIS) provided to parents at the time of immunizations. Don't you think it should be?

Safety: On the flip side, many of us know that, according to the FDA, vaccines are not 100 percent safe. Any medications we take carry potential risks. Just as effectiveness varies for each vaccine, safety profiles also vary for each vaccine. Not all vaccinations are created equal and one vaccination may have more associated adverse reactions (side effects) than others. For example, the CDC's Vaccine Adverse Events Reporting System (VAERS) reports that the diphtheria, tetanus, and pertussis (DTaP) vaccination has one of the higher numbers of reported adverse reactions, while varicella (chicken pox) has one of the lower numbers of reported adverse reactions. It is important to be informed about each separate vaccination, what it contains, and its individual risks and benefits prior to vaccinating. Many helpful resources to assist you can be found in the Resource Guide in Part 3 or at www.behindcloseddoorsthebook.com.

In an honest attempt to bring both sides of the vaccine issue closer together and as mothers, we need to understand and respect one thing—each of our experiences with vaccinations may be different. Here are two different experiences with a vaccine reaction.

AN ADVERSE REACTION TAKEN SERIOUSLY (JOANNE)

When we drove home from my son Colin's four-month well visit, he was fast asleep. When he awoke an hour later, I knew something wasn't right. He persisted with a high-pitched cry that couldn't be consoled. I tried walking, burping, feeding, and changing. I took off all his clothes just to be certain nothing was sticking or poking him. For hours we paced and cried together, and I called the doctor's office twice. The nurses could hear his cry over the phone, and I was told that my son was most likely experiencing an adverse reaction to the DTP (diphtheria, tetanus toxoids, and whole-cell pertussis) shot he'd just received. The crying slowly settled as a result of complete exhaustion, around the seven-hour mark, and he then slept for nearly twelve hours, much longer than normal.

We followed up with the pediatrician and were instructed that Colin was not to ever receive the "pertussis" component of the DTP vaccine again. My pediatrician said he'd already reported the reaction to VAERS. Our nurse that day was incredible and emphatic with me about understanding the importance of what we were being told.

"You may move from this practice someday," she said, "and although it will be written in Colin's chart, as his mother you will be his last line of defense at the time of immunizations. Anytime anyone steps into the room to give any immunizations, you check and double-check that none contains pertussis."

Looking back, I realize how fortunate I was to have found such as a great pediatric practice. My pediatrician at that time handled the serious adverse reaction exactly how it was supposed to be handled and made sure Colin was medically exempt due to his reaction. The nurse empowered me to feel free to question anyone putting anything into my child's body. Years later, with drug safety experience under my belt, I now fully understand that it wasn't the high-pitched persistent crying that was the problem. That was just the reported symptom. The real problem (and reason for the crying) was most likely brain swelling that can sometimes result in permanent neurological damage. Although Colin did experience speech and language delays and other early learning problems, the outcome could have been much worse if my doctor had not been so vigilant in responding to the reaction the way he did.

EVERY PARENT'S STORY MATTERS (CHRISTINE)

While at a children's play gym my sister and I met a woman and her autistic son. We started making small talk and it turned out that we'd shared the same pediatrician and each of us had spent a lot of time there. I tried to acknowledge all the hardships I could only assume she'd faced on a daily basis after receiving her son's diagnosis of autism. I also shared my struggles with Kaleigh, which seemed small in comparison. As I did, she began to open up about her son's diagnosis.

"On the way home from the doctor's office after several immunizations in one day," she said, "my son started shaking uncontrollably in his car seat. When I called the doctor to report the symptoms, I was told that my son was 'just cold' and that it was not related to the shots he had just received. From that point on, it was like 'the lights went out' in my son and we eventually received a diagnosis of autism. In my gut, I believe that the shots were responsible, but our pediatrician refused to acknowledge this."

My sister and I could see how upsetting this recollection of events was to the woman and we immediately said, "We believe you."

The mother's eyes filled with gratitude.

"You believe me?" she asked.

"Yes," we said again, "we believe you."

Her entire demeanor changed, as if she was relieved that what had happened to her son wasn't being dismissed yet again. Her story mattered and her son mattered. All we'd done was taken the time to listen and understand and validate what she believed happened to her son."

Vaccine Adverse Events Reporting System (VAERS)

According to the CDC, a large part of our vaccine safety information comes from the general population through postmarketing safety surveillance and adverse event reporting following vaccines. There are approximately 30,000 vaccine reaction reports filed annually in the United States, with 10–15 percent of those classified as *serious* (resulting in permanent disability, birth defect, hospitalization, life-threatening illnesses, or death). The CDC reports that most adverse reactions are mild and will resolve without injury. Additionally, it's important to note that *not* every adverse reaction reported is believed to be associated with the vaccination.

But it's also important to note that the system doctors and parents are encouraged to use to report vaccine reactions—the CDC's Vaccine Adverse Events Reporting System (VAERS)—is by the admission of the FDA and CDC, a *passive* system. Simply put, the very reporting system we use and heavily rely on for safety data is grossly underutilized. Although the FDA requires doctors and other vaccine providers to report to VAERS hospitalizations, injuries, deaths, and serious health problems following vaccination, there are no legal sanctions against doctors for *not* reporting a reaction; it's estimated that only about 10 percent of the *actual* adverse events associated with vaccines are ever reported. So although only 30,000 adverse reaction reports are estimated to be filed each year, that may be only a *small percentage* of the real number of adverse reactions children actually experience. This highlights a real problem. One reason VAERS remains a passive system is partly because many parents are unaware of reactions that vaccines may cause.

Although parents are usually made aware of potential immediate vaccine reactions, we're not being made aware of *all* the possible reactions including delayed reactions and the correlation between various symptoms and possible long-term health effects. For instance, while we may recognize a seizure to be a serious neurological side effect of a vaccine, many of us may not grasp that difficulty with waking a baby, vomiting, or a high-pitched, persistent cry immediately following a vaccination *may* also be the sign of a neurological side effect caused by brain inflammation (known as encephalitis). Although most cases of encephalitis are mild with full recovery, when prolonged it can lead to damage of the brain tissue, developmental problems, learning disabilities, and other serious health issues that don't surface until months or years later.

If we don't use VAERS the way it was intended—reporting all *potential* adverse reactions from vaccines so they can be evaluated as such—then the *safety profile* of the vaccine will remain unaffected. We also need VAERS and other vaccine surveillance systems to monitor for long-term health outcomes, as some of the science suggests a connection between vaccines and autoimmune disorders that don't surface until a few months following vaccines.

Parents are encouraged by the CDC to report any possible reactions they observe to VAERS. For more information on reporting adverse reactions to VAERS and other information on this searchable database of vaccine reactions, see the Resource Guide in Part 3 or at www. behindcloseddoorsthebook.com.

[Authors' note: Although encephalitis is a known potential side effect from vaccinations, it is also a side effect of some of the diseases that vaccines can prevent. The most well-documented example of an autoimmune disorder reaction to a vaccine noted in the paragraph above was an outbreak of Guillain-Barré syndrome in 1976– 1977, as a result of a swine flu vaccine campaign.]

Vaccine Information Sheets

Many parents are under the assumption that the Vaccine Information Sheets (VIS) provided at the time a vaccination is administered contains full disclosure of vaccine risks and benefits. This is *not* the case. Vaccine Information Sheets (VIS) were developed to fulfill information requirements under the National Childhood Vaccine Injury Act. They are *not* considered *informed consent* forms, which would have to provide all the benefits and all the risks and also allow every person the right to refusal. Although VIS provides parents with important and accurate information, VIS fails to inform us of the vaccine ingredients, the expected rate of effectiveness of the vaccine, and a complete list of all the adverse events associated with the vaccine's clinical trials and postmarketing safety surveillance. Do you think we have a right to know how effective the vaccine is, or if an ingredient, such as aluminum, is in any of the vaccines our child is scheduled to receive? Do you think we also have the right to know *cumulative levels* of any potentially toxic ingredients when *multiple vaccines* are given in one day? Although the VIS has undergone some major improvements of late, is more balanced and complete information still needed?

Vaccine Courts, Taxes, and Immunity for the Pharmaceutical Industry

Pharmaceutical companies were granted *immunity* from most lawsuits resulting from vaccine injuries or deaths under the National Childhood Vaccine Injury Act of 1986. The Act was established in part because costly lawsuits were affecting the price and availability of vaccines and in part because government officials acknowledged that a small percent of infants and children can suffer severe reactions leading to permanent disability or death. As a result, The National Vaccine Injury Compensation Program was created to compensate vaccine-related injuries or deaths from recommended vaccinations (sometimes referred to as "vaccine courts"). The program was established as a *no-fault* alternative to the traditional tort system for resolving vaccine injury claims. In other words, the vaccine manufacturers are not being held "accountable for" or "at fault for" the damages their vaccines may cause.

Instead, *we* pay into the compensation settlements through a special *vaccine excise tax* paid at the time our child receives any of the CDC recommended immunizations. Each vaccine dose requires a separate tax. For example, the MMR vaccine is taxed three times because it's administered for three diseases. This tax speaks volumes about the potential risks, yet we aren't being told up front that we must pay this surcharge. Why? Money from this tax goes into the *Vaccine Injury Compensation Trust Fund* set up to compensate infants, children, and adults. The U.S. Court of Federal Claims ultimately decides who will receive payments due to injuries or death associated with a vaccine. Vaccine settlements from the fund have reached *3.5 billion dollars* since claims began in 1989—after the vaccine manufacturers received immunity. According to a 2015 statistical report from the Department of Health and Human Services, the most compensation award money has been granted to injuries or death from pertussis-containing vaccines and influenza vaccines.

It's troubling that vaccine manufacturers aren't being held fully accountable for the safety of their product. Surely the car industry would be held accountable if a car malfunction caused death or disability. Where is a manufacturer's motivation to make improvements in safety? We are the only country in the world where one can't bring a lawsuit against a pharmaceutical company for damages from a vaccine and have a jury of our peers decide the verdict.

The U.S. Department of Health and Human Services Health Resources and Services Administration (HRSA) website lists and explains injuries/conditions presumed to be caused by vaccines. It also details the time periods in which the first symptom of these injuries/conditions must occur after receiving the vaccine to be eligible for compensation under the National Childhood Vaccine Injury Act of 1986. More information on the table of presumed injuries caused by vaccinations can be found in Resource Guide in Part 3 or at www.behindcloseddoorsthebook.com.

[Authors' note: The compensation program originated to provide a fast, less traumatic, and less costly alternative to a lawsuit for those injured. However, critics feel it has evolved into a lengthy, challenging process with increasingly stricter guidelines for compensation.]

Vaccine Requirement Laws

Vaccine policies are made at the federal level, but vaccine laws are made at the state level. Vaccine laws and requirements differ from state to state, but *every* state allows you to waive any vaccine for *medical reasons*—which require a doctor's note. All states (with the exception of California, Mississippi, and West Virginia) allow you to waive vaccines for *religious beliefs*. Fifteen states allow you to decline vaccines for philosophical reasons.

Today, more and more states are introducing legislation to take away the right to waive vaccines for reasons other than medical. This raises important points to consider such as the following: Do state governments have the right to mandate something that has the potential to cause permanent disability or even death? Should vaccinations require true informed consent like all other medical procedures in our country? Is it a Constitutional right to decide what we put into our bodies and the bodies of our children? Or, is it our *civic responsibility* to vaccinate, regardless of the known risks and potential for harm, to protect the greater good of all? For information about vaccination in your state, see the Resource Guide in Part 3 or at www.behindcloseddoorsthebook.com.

Do Your Own Research:
Spend Time Examining Both Sides of the Debate

It is well worth the time to look into the research behind any statements made to support either side of the vaccine debate. It is important to note that there are many highly respected medical journals with published studies supporting *both* the relative safety of vaccines and the potential for harm from vaccines. As consumers of health information it is helpful if we can learn how to be a critical reader and look closely at things that can influence a study. Some important points to note are: Who has funded the study we are examining? Do conflicts of interest exist? What type of study design was used? This is a biggie, because different types of studies are subject to different types of bias. Data obtained from randomized controlled trials are considered the "gold standard" for evidence of safety and efficacy. Another important point to consider is, whether the study was published in a peer-reviewed journal. Peer-reviewed journal articles are considered to have the greatest integrity and hold the most scientific value because they have a system of checks and balances incorporated into their methodology—including bipartisan (unbiased) reviewers. We encourage you to do your own vaccine research and closely review any vaccine studies you choose to take value from. The bottom line is that the study headlines you read or study sound bites you hear will not disclose many of these very important underlying details.

Did You Know?

Pharmaceutical companies and government agencies charged with vaccine oversight often hire public relations management firms. Naturally, all public relations campaigns are carefully designed to affect how vaccine information is delivered in the news. Pharmaceutical *advertising* dollars also directly *fund* the media and can strongly influence what we hear about vaccines in a news outlet, and—what we don't.

CAUGHT IN THE MIDDLE (SUE D., CRNP)

I have been a nurse practitioner for twelve years and for eight of those years I have worked in a family practice seeing infants and children for their well exams that always included ordering immunizations appropriate for their ages. During graduate school I learned about vaccinations, their origins, their uses, and the diseases they prevented. At the time, I was confident that all the information I had been provided regarding vaccinations would prepare me to answer any questions that would arise in my practice.

I soon found out that I was not ready to handle specific questions regarding vaccine safety, conflicts of interest, long-term studies, and vaccine-injured children that I received from concerned parents during visits, as well as from friends and family. If the truth be told, my ego was also slightly bruised because I couldn't always provide an immediate answer. When first approached with questions on these topics, my natural reaction was to tell people that vaccines are absolutely safe and that they had been "misinformed" somewhere along the line (often thinking silently to myself that they were crazy to even question vaccine safety). In my mind, if any of the concerns they raised were truly valid, as a healthcare provider, I would have been informed about them somewhere along the line. However, as a healthcare provider (and mother myself) I felt obliged to swallow my pride and check into the safety concerns that had been brought to my attention.

After spending a lot of time looking through medical journals and other peer-reviewed publications, I was quite humbled by many of my findings. It surprised me that I was not receiving more balanced information as a healthcare provider. Although I found many studies to support vaccine safety, I also found many studies that questioned it. Some scientists are very concerned that immunizations may be affecting the immune health of our children and have recommended further safety studies. Additionally, like many other healthcare providers, I was unaware that our government had set up a compensation program for vaccine-injured children and adults. Unfortunately, serious vaccine injuries do occur and there needs to be more research on why certain children are more biologically susceptible to injuries so improvement to identify such children prior to vaccinating can be made. Increased efforts to provide more balanced vaccine information to healthcare providers can help us more confidently and more honestly address parental concerns.

I now understand why some parents have raised concern about various aspects of our vaccine program. Although I feel strongly that the practice of vaccinating against serious diseases is very important, some safety questions surrounding the cumulative effects of the schedule and possible long-term health outcomes remain largely unanswered.

Vaccines are a heated issue with anger and frustration on both sides. I know many healthcare providers feel like their backs are thrown against the wall when they are drilled with questions they are unprepared to answer in the ten minutes they are allotted to see patients. And parents with valid concerns feel ostracized for raising questions about ingredients or the recommended schedule. Instead of taking sides, we should all be working together to encourage improvements and safeguards in our vaccine policies that support better communication among the federal agencies providing vaccine oversight, healthcare providers, and parents. We also need to conduct well-designed research studies that can be replicated, including studies that evaluate the safety of our current childhood immunization schedule as well as the long-term health outcomes the schedule is producing. And most importantly, if we want these studies to hold validity for everyone involved they should be conducted by an independent party so that confidence and trust in the vaccination program can once again be restored.

Encouraging News about Vaccines

It is important to reiterate that this chapter did not share the many benefits of vaccines. We only highlighted areas of concern that lack transparency and may have potentially contributed to the increases over the past few decades in many children's chronic health issues. Understanding both the benefits and the risks is equally important. We have included in our Resource Guide (see Part 3 or www.behindcloseddoorsthebook.com) many government websites that you can access for additional information on vaccine benefits.

This may have been the first time you learned of any associated risks or conflict of interests regarding our vaccine program. As mothers and parents, first learning about these issues can evoke an array of uncomfortable emotions including feelings of guilt and anger. It is worth stating again that no matter what our stance is on vaccines, as parents, we only have the best interest of our children at heart when making health decisions.

Vaccine Practical Tools

✓ *Vaccine Brand Choice*: It is empowering to know that sometimes more than one manufacturer makes the same vaccination and often uses different vaccine ingredients. For example, one brand may contain aluminum while another brand of the same vaccine does not contain aluminum. This can be very helpful to parents who are concerned about vaccine ingredients that are potentially toxic to the brain (such as thimerosal and aluminum) or contain ingredients their children may be allergic to (such as egg) but still want the benefits of vaccinations. By knowing your brand choices and knowing what ingredients are in each of your child's vaccines, you can vaccinate more confidently. Ask your healthcare provider about your brand choices and the ingredient differences before you vaccinate. They may have to order a specific brand in for you or let you know where one is available. Helpful websites that allow you to quickly and easily explore different brand choices and ingredients are discussed next and are also included in our Resource Guide in Part 3 or at www.behindcloseddoorsthebook.com.

✓ *Vaccine Ingredients Calculator*: If you are concerned about vaccine ingredients or just want to examine all your manufacturer brand choices before you vaccinate, this empowering, interactive web tool of The National Vaccine Information Center can help. When you enter your child's age and weight and then choose the age-appropriate vaccinations recommended by the CDC, your child's vaccine brand options appear. You can then compare the major ingredients in each manufacturer's vaccine and choose the brand that you feel most comfortable with for your child. The Vaccine Ingredients Calculator also allows you to keep track of just how much of certain ingredients your child may be exposed to in each separate vaccine and will automatically warn you if any ingredient exceeds any established safety standards set for that ingredient based on your child's weight. It will also warn you if any combinations of vaccines planned for the same day cumulatively exceed any established safety standards for your child's weight. If safer options are available through a different vaccine brand it will alert you. You can then discuss these findings with your healthcare provider. This tool provides parents concerned with vaccine ingredients full transparency as well as greater confidence when vaccinating. See the Resource Guide for more information. *[Authors' note: The FDA and CDC do not make any recommendations to dose vaccines by weight. This tool is merely providing consumers additional transparency into the combined and cumulative amounts of vaccine ingredients a child may be exposed to at a single visit and any safety concerns that may be associated with these levels for their body weight. For example, it may reference a safety standard set by the EPA for an ingredient like ethylmercury that is based on weight.]*

✓ *Manufacturer's Package Inserts:* The most complete and reliable source of information available to us on any vaccination can be found in the manufacturers package inserts of each separate vaccine. We encourage you to read these before vaccinating. Full prescribing inserts will contain important information regarding drug interactions, contraindications, adverse reactions, warnings, precautions, ingredients, and effectiveness not commonly found on the vaccine information sheets (VIS) provided by your healthcare provider at the time of each vaccine. Vaccine package inserts should be made available to view wherever your child receives their vaccinations and are also available online to review on the website of the FDA. More information can be found in the Resource Guide. *[Authors' note: Although patients may obtain useful information from these inserts, its primary purpose is to give healthcare professionals the information they need to prescribe drugs appropriately.]*

✓ *Boosting the Immune System to Prevent Vaccine Reactions*: According to the 2013 Institute of Medicine (IOM) report, children with healthy immune systems are less likely to suffer a serious vaccine reaction. Robert W. Sears, MD, FAAP, a board-certified pediatrician and coauthor of several books in the Sears parenting library, advocates for boosting your child's immune system prior to vaccinations. According to Dr. Sears, "Most vaccine side effects involve the immune system reacting poorly to the vaccine, so insuring a healthy immune system is one way parents can decrease their child's risk of a vaccine reaction." Here are some of his suggestions: breastfeed, minimize sugar and junk food, minimize chemical exposure, eat fruits and vegetables, and assure adequate amounts of omega-3 oil supplements, probiotics, Vitamin A, and Vitamin C. See the Resource Guide for more details.

✓ *Alternative Vaccine Schedules*: There are several books written by pediatricans that discuss alternative vaccine schedules as an option for parents concerned about the rigor of our current schedule and potential adverse reactions. Alternative vaccine schedules often suggest only giving one vaccine at a time and spreading the vaccines out over longer periods of time. Some even suggest delaying vaccinations until twelve months of age when the immune system is more mature. The bottom line is that a growing number of parents want options. If healthcare providers do not work with parents to provide more flexibility, more parents may choose to opt out of vaccines altogether (where state laws allow this). Most healthcare providers would rather have you vaccinate at a slower pace than not vaccinate at all. For more information on alternative schedules see the Resource Guide. *[Authors' note: Alternative schedules are obviously **not endorsed** by the CDC.]*

✓ *Titer Testing*: A blood test known as a "titer" is another valuable tool for vaccine-sensitive children. The test measures the level of antibodies someone has acquired in their body to help fight a certain disease. Antibodies can derive from natural exposure to a disease or from a vaccination. Information from this blood test can help to determine if a child needs a vaccination or not. Some doctors who practice environmental medicine use titer testing prior to scheduled vaccinations in children who seem to be very susceptible to toxic overload. It is theorized that if booster shots (any repeat doses of a vaccine after the initial shot) are given before needed, immune overload can result in certain populations of children, leading to a variety of health effects. For example, Joanne's niece, Kate, was quite sensitive to various environmental toxins as an infant and toddler, so as a precaution her pediatrician ordered vaccine titer tests to see if Kate's body was ready for, or in need of the vaccine booster shots. From this test, it was determined that Kate still had high levels of antibodies (protection) from her previous vaccines, two years and counting after she was due for her booster shots according to the vaccine schedule. This is a perfect example of how a one-size-fits-all vaccine program is not always effective for every child. Titer testing can be a valuable tool to use in certain populations of children and may even help prevent some potential vaccine reactions.

With all our children are exposed to these days, we may have unknowingly created a perfect storm not only for our children but also for the vaccine program so many have faith in. U.S. children can receive twenty-five vaccine doses before their first birthday and fifty vaccine doses before their first day of kindergarten. What we are questioning is if the vaccine protocols our children are subjected to—never intended to bring harm upon any child, only intended as a means to protect them—may just be the tipping point for the developing bodies of some children. Once again, it all adds up.

It is important to reiterate that we are not taking a stance for or against vaccinations. We are only taking a stand for our right as parents and citizens to have more balanced information and true informed consent at the time of vaccinations. It is not about being provaccine, antivaccine, or somewhere in the middle. It is about standing together as parents and protectors of our children to ensure that every single state-mandated vaccine is truly warranted and mandated free from conflicts of interest. It is about demanding independent long-term vaccine safety studies so parents can have greater confidence in the system. And it is about rethinking our one-size-fits-all program. We need to find a middle ground where we can all recognize the need for some level of vaccine reforms and begin to work together to create the changes that will ensure better health and safety for *all* our children.

Section 5: Mental Health Treatment Trends

> *I met the mother of a 29-month-old boy who wanted me to prescribe*
> *medication. I didn't, but later I learned the boy was getting lithium,*
> *Zoloft, and Risperdal from another doctor. . . . Is this cutting-edge*
> *treatment or an outrage? I am not sure.*
> —Lawrence H. Diller, MD, Pediatric Behavioral Psychiatrist
> from "Kids on Drugs," published by Salon Media Group

OBSERVATIONS ON CURRENT TRENDS
(SCOTT SHANNON, MD, CHILD AND ADOLESCENT PSYCHIATRIST)

Mental health issues for American children grow more distressing every year. For example, the rates of depression, anxiety, ADHD, and autism have increased in each ensuing decade over the last half-century. Sadly, only one out of every four or five of these struggling children ever find any type of treatment. We can speculate why our children's mental health is failing: more stress, poor nutrition, less sleep, inadequate exercise, electronic overstimulation, greater levels of obesity, etc. However, we are left with one harsh reality—it is difficult to find treatment for these increasingly common problems.

Child psychiatrists are pressed to address these issues. Unfortunately, mine is the most underserved subspecialty in all of medicine with less than 8,000 docs trying to meet the demand, when over 40,000 child psychiatrists are needed. As a result, professionals feel pushed to the point of desperation: child psychiatrists often prescribe medications quickly, without adequate evidence for safety or effectiveness. Conversely, most parents feel stressed with this process and frequently there is no discussion about proven nonmedication options for their child's mental health. Parents must become empowered to understand the breadth of options available for their child. Finally, all of us need to become engaged and work towards true support for the sound mental health of our young people.

We have seen from the statistics in Chapter 3 that mental health disorders in our nation's children have increased dramatically over the past few decades. Over the same time period, the use of psychiatric drugs to treat these disorders has skyrocketed. For some children, psychiatric drugs such as antidepressants, antianxiety agents, stimulants, mood stabilizers, and antipsychotics have provided good results and will play a vital and necessary role in improving the child's quality of life. Other children have found greater success in alternative therapies (e.g., behavioral or talk or nutritional therapies) that allow either a lower dose of a drug or a completely drug-free therapy. There is no one-size-fits-all answer to mental health—and there likely never will be. Each child is unique and as parents we need to work with our healthcare provider to find the formula that works best for our child and our personal situation.

With that being said, there are many concerns about the ever-growing number of children and teens taking psychiatric drugs. The long-term effects of medicating children with mind- and mood-altering drugs during their developmental years are largely unknown. But the younger the child, the more potentially devastating the effects may be on the developing brain. The drug side effects can potentially be so serious that many carry "black box" warning labels—the most serious warning the FDA issues.

Especially concerning is the use of one type of psychiatric drug, *antipsychotics,* in some of our nation's youngest children. Antipsychotics (such as Risperdal and Seroquel) are primarily used to treat disorders such as schizophrenia and bipolar disorder. However, recently there has been a trend in prescribing these drugs to children for indications (such as ADHD) and in age groups (such as toddlers)—that have *not been tested and FDA approved* (known as "off-label" uses). Over the last ten to fifteen years, the use of antipsychotic drugs in U.S. children has tripled with younger and younger children being prescribed this serious class of medication with a long list of potential side effects that include: *a loss of brain volume, excessive weight gain, an increased risk of diabetes, increased cholesterol, rapid heartbeat that may lead to sudden death, movement disorders, increased prolactin levels (hormonal changes), and the development of breast tissue in boys.*

Another area of concern is that many of these antipsychotic drugs are being prescribed increasingly by pediatricians—not psychiatrists. The American Academy of Pediatrics says that these medications (given their serious risks) should be a treatment of last resort. However, this is not always what happens. According to child and adolescent psychiatrist Dr. Scott Shannon, "Doctors are increasingly pulled along by desperation of parents, cultural expectations, and a lack of knowledge about other nonpharma options."

A 2010 study published in the *Journal of the American Academy of Child & Adolescent Psychiatry* revealed that *fewer* than *one-half* of antipsychotic-treated young children between the ages of two and five ever received a mental health assessment (40.8 percent), a psychotherapy visit (41.4 percent), or a visit with a psychiatrist (42.6 percent) during the year of antipsychotic use. This is concerning because a mental health provider will not only provide a careful mental health assessment, but explore various other types of interventions first, before resorting to medications with serious side effects. For example, behavioral interventions and talk therapies often uncover triggers to a child's behaviors and give a child a sense of control over their emotions. Exploring common stressors such as inadequate nutrition, unaddressed trauma, learning problems, family relationships, and more can also identify the root of behavioral and emotional issues.

One large barrier to providing more *balanced* treatment options to young children is that mental health practitioners and alternative therapies are not always *accessible* or *affordable* to all children. Our shortage of child and adolescent psychiatrists highlights this problem. Shouldn't it be a national healthcare priority that young children being medicated with powerful psychiatric drugs be under the care of a mental health provider? And that all children have access to drug-free therapy options?

It's not uncommon for a young child with ADHD or another behavioral health disorder to be taking more than one mood- or mind-altering medication at the same time. A child with ADHD may be on a stimulant medication (such as Adderall) along with an antipsychotic (such as Risperdal). And when side effects from either one of these psychoactive medications arise, they are sometimes given *additional* medication to offset them. Before you know it a young child can be on a cocktail of different medications for a growing list of medical problems. Is this practice in balance?

NIXING THE PRESCRIPTION QUICK FIX (MARY)

By age five, my daughter Kate, was making great strides in many of her behaviors related to autism. My husband and I took her to a pediatric specialist who said that his only remaining concern was Kate's social development. The doctor suggested a common ADHD drug, Ritalin, to help with her social interactions. She was on Ritalin for two weeks and went from being a bubbly child to a withdrawn girl with no clue about what was going on around her, but hyperfocused on the task at hand. Due to her reaction, the doctor then suggested we replace Ritalin with an antihypertension drug, Tenex, used to lower blood pressure in adults. We tried it for a month but unfortunately Kate's behavior became more aggressive and erratic, escalating to a horrifying point when she exclaimed, "I just want to kill myself." All her doctor could say was that this was likely a side effect from the Tenex.

He then suggested adding Risperdal, an antipsychotic drug, to deal with the side effects of Tenex. By now we were panicked at the thought of our five-year-old daughter taking a powerful mind-altering drug just to improve her social interactions. We refused to continue the pharmaceutical treatment, but pursued alternative therapies, including environmental medicine and dietary interventions that addressed Kate's food sensitivities that often impacted her behaviors. While this was not a quick-fix approach, we were far more comfortable with it, and for Kate it eventually proved to hold much better results without the risk of unknown and potentially harmful side effects.

In 2015, the CDC released its first-ever national ADHD treatment study showing that 25 percent of U.S. *preschoolers* taking ADHD medications were doing so without having tried behavioral interventions first. The CDC found this concerning because the long-term effects of psychotropic medications on the developing mind and bodies of young children are unknown. According to the CDC, behavioral therapy is safe and can have long-term positive benefits on how a child with ADHD functions at home, at school, and with friends. The American Academy of Pediatrics recommends *behavioral therapy* as the first line of treatment for ADHD in children under age six.

The growing number of children on psychiatric drugs is a concerning topic that deserves to be addressed. Although we were only able to touch on this topic due to limited space and the complexity of the problem, we pose some questions for you to consider in regard to current trends that need may need reform:

- Are mental health services and drug-free therapy options available and accessible to all children?
- Are doctor's receiving and sharing information about nonpharma options with parents?
- Are parents and teens well informed of the serious side effects of individual and combined drug therapies?
- Can drug therapy be contributing to additional health problems in our children?
- Are we working to identify the root cause of mental and behavioral health problems?

[Authors' note: Atypical antipsychotic drugs have side effects that can vary from child to child and by the individual drug. The FDA has approved two antipsychotics (risperidone and aripiprazole) to treat behavioral problems and irritability in children diagnosed with autism aged five to seventeen. Antipsychotics are not approved for use in autistic children under the age of five.]

Did You Know?

 Antipsychotics are now one of the biggest moneymakers for the U.S. pharmaceutical industry, with sales growing from $3 billion dollars a year in 2003 to an estimated $18 billion today. This success may have been in part due to illegal marketing tactics used to get these profitable medications into the hands of our nation's children for indications and in age groups never approved by the FDA. In 2013, one of our country's largest pharmaceutical companies paid over a billion dollars to settle allegations for illegal and aggressive marketing of an antipsychotic drug to doctors and pharmacists on behalf of the ever-growing number of U.S. children with ADHD and other behavioral disorders. Allegations included providing false statements about the drug's safety and efficacy, as well as paying kickbacks to doctors for prescribing the drug. Although it's perfectly legal for healthcare providers to prescribe drugs for off-label uses, it remains highly illegal for drug makers to promote their products for any purpose not approved by the FDA or to make false or misleading statements regarding a products safety or efficacy.

---

*[**Important note:** It could be dangerous to immediately stop taking a psychiatric drug due to potentially significant withdrawal side effects. Please do not ever stop taking any psychiatric drug without the advice and assistance of a competent healthcare provider.]*

ENCOURAGING NEWS FROM A TEACHER (CATHY, FIFTH-GRADE TEACHER)

The one positive change I have seen in my profession recently is that parents and students are more health conscientious. Twenty years ago there was a big push from parents (and teachers) to place kids on medications for certain learning and behavioral problems. Today, I see a growing number of parents working with teachers in an effort to use the least amount of medication possible by taking a closer look at some outside influences on the problem. Just by monitoring the foods their children are eating parents have made a difference in their children's ability to concentrate in the classroom.

Practical Tools for Mental Health

See the Resource Guide in Part 3 or at www.behindcloseddoors thebook.com for additional information and practical tools related to behavioral and mental health issues.

Chapter 7

THE ENVIRONMENT

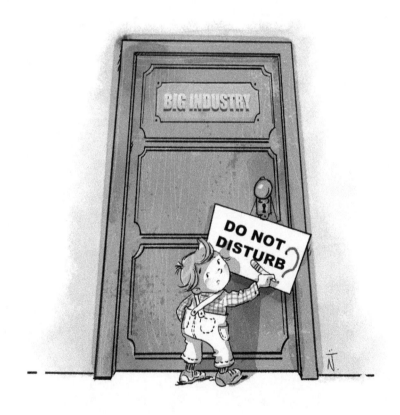

In our way of life, in our government, with every decision we make,
we always keep in mind the Seventh Generation to come. It's our job
to see that the people coming ahead, the generations still unborn,
have a world no worse than ours and hopefully better.
—Oren Lyons, an Iroquois tribal leader

SEARCHING FOR ANSWERS, MAKING CONNECTIONS (JOANNE)

In 1992, Patrick started a new school and I got to know one of the moms at the bus stop. She had grown up in the area and when I mentioned my concerns about environmental factors in the development of Patrick's brain tumor, she asked if I was familiar with the Salford Quarry Superfund site about a mile away. I told her no, but that I'd look into it. A Superfund site is any land that has been contaminated by hazardous waste and identified by the EPA as a candidate for cleanup because it poses a risk to the health of people or the environment.

I went to the library and sifted through all the information related to our local Superfund site (this information could not be checked out, but was kept in a special room). After spending hours poring over numerous binders, I began making some connections between this environment and cancer. A shale quarry from the early 1900s was later used as a dumping ground, circa the 1950s, for industrial, commercial, and residential waste. A tile company then purchased the land and used it for getting rid of glaze sludge, scrap tiles, and other waste. In 1982, two 10,000-gallon tanks containing boron and fuel oil were found buried on the site. According to the EPA, on- and off-site groundwater had been contaminated with large amounts of boron as well as volatile organic compounds, such as trichloroethylene or TCE, 1-2-dichloroethene, and vinyl chloride (chemical components of solvents and degreasers), along with inorganic metals such as lead. Some of these substances were known or suspected to cause cancer.

The contaminated groundwater threatened both private wells and municipal wells that carried water to homes and businesses.

Approximately 54,000 people were drawing drinking water from wells within three miles of the site. In 1987, the EPA began addressing the boron contamination by shutting down the municipal well closest to the site and ensured that all nearby residents with well water were hooked up to public water.

The old quarry Superfund site was now on the EPA's National Priority List (NPL), making it a top concern among all Superfund sites across the country and allocating funds for its cleanup. The EPA still needed to address the source of the contamination, as waste remained buried on-site that could further contaminate the groundwater.

At the library, I found minutes from community meetings revealing how local residents were also worried that their children may have been exposed to a number of these toxins as they played or fished in a nearby creek. The minutes also gave personal accounts of illness and cancers in some residents in close proximity to the site. I came away from this research with a heightened awareness of the cause and effect of environmental contaminants. I also felt empowered. While it was upsetting to learn about an EPA Superfund site in my community, knowing about it gave me some sense of control. It was reassuring to learn that the EPA was involved in overseeing its cleanup and that all the wells in close proximity to the site had been shut down.

I now saw the relevance of the questions the staff from the epidemiology department at Children's Hospital of Philadelphia had asked my husband and me after Patrick's surgery. Where did we live? Where did I grow up? Did we live near a farm? My mind raced back to my childhood hometown, where so many neighbors on my street had died prematurely from cancer. Now my son had been diagnosed with a cancerous brain tumor. Was there a connection to an environmental problem there?

The development where my parents purchased a home in the early 1960s was built on farmland, and I often wondered if a chemical pesticide like DDT had been used there. DDT is likely to cause cancer in humans and does not break down easily in the environment. It can also be released into the air or seep into the soil and eventually make its way into groundwater, potentially contaminating drinking water from public or private wells. DDT can remain in the human body for decades after exposure.

Growing up there were also rumors of "buried" toxic waste and various "testing" from two nearby military operations located within three miles on either side of our development. Was there any truth to this? Were there toxic dump sites like the quarry in the area where I grew up?

Section 1: Body Burden

If you want to learn about the health of a population, look at the air they breathe, the water they drink, and the places where they live.
—Hippocrates, the Father of Medicine, fifth century B.C.

The environment directly affects our health as humans —and most especially the health of our children. This simple concept is one that many of us are just now beginning to fully understand. As humans we rely on the environment for survival. We get our oxygen, our water, our food, and our shelter from the environment. So when we contaminate the environment with pollution and toxic chemicals, it should be common sense that we are really just contaminating ourselves in the process. If the environment is not healthy, humans will not be healthy, and our children will not thrive. It really is that simple.

The health effects of a toxic environment are often first seen in the youngest creatures living in that environment. Our children's health statistics over the past few decades surely support this notion. As we continually increase the number of toxic chemicals we put into our environment and our homes, we continually compromise the health of our infants and children. There's mounting scientific evidence linking many environmental toxins to a host of chronic illnesses, diseases, and neurological problems in our children including cancer, birth defects, learning disabilities, developmental delays, hyperactivity, autism, asthma, allergies, obesity, diabetes, rheumatoid arthritis, and early puberty. Pollution is not just something the *earth* is experiencing, but something we're *all* experiencing. Studies have demonstrated just how vulnerable we are to exposure and how infants and children are the most unprotected of all.

Did You Know?

 The Environmental Working Group (EWG) is one of our nation's leading environmental health research and advocacy organizations (nonprofit). Its mission is to conduct original, game-changing research that inspires people, businesses, and governments to take action to protect human health and the environment.

Over the past twelve years, the Environmental Working Group (EWG) and the CDC have conducted extensive research on chemical pollution *in the bodies* of American people. These are known as "body burden" studies. The EWG alone has tested more than 200 Americans for 540 different industrial chemicals and found up to 482 of the chemicals present in the blood and urine of those examined.

Of all the studies done, none has had a more profound effect than when the EWG took its body burden research one step farther. The EWG wanted to see if our *unborn babies* were protected from the same industrial chemicals, pollutants, and pesticides adults were vulnerable to. In 2004, the EWG followed ten pregnant mothers and subsequently their *newborn* American babies. According to EWG president Ken Cook, "This was the first time anyone had ever bothered, since the beginning of the chemical revolution, to examine umbilical cord blood to see how many toxic chemicals got through to the developing child." What they discovered was sobering. Researchers found, on average, 200 *industrial chemicals* present in the *umbilical cord blood* of these newborn babies, proving that these infants were exposed to *toxic* chemicals *in utero*. Developing babies were also being exposed to a host of *everyday* chemicals that their mothers were exposed to, including dioxins and furans, heavy metals, flame retardants, BPA, perchlorate (rocket fuel component), nonstick or "Teflon-like" chemicals, and various other active ingredients in common household products, personal care products, and industrial pollution. Even more disturbing was that these newborn babies were also found to be contaminated with chemicals and pesticides *banned* over thirty years earlier—including lead, PCBs, and the pesticide DDT—chemicals that were *still pervasive* in our environment.

The chemicals detected in these newborn babies are known to cause cancer as well as other neurological, endocrine, and immune system disruptions, which could lead to learning disabilities, developmental delays, and various other health conditions many of our children are now experiencing. All of this exposure took place *before* these ten newborns ever took their first breath. This powerful study made headline news because it could potentially explain and maybe even help prevent many health issues our children are currently suffering from.

This study highlighted the full impact of weak safety standards for chemicals and the critical role our environment plays in our children's health. In April 2010, President Obama's Cancer Panel declared that "to a disturbing extent, babies are being born 'pre-polluted'" and that "there is a critical lack of knowledge and appreciation of environmental threats to children's health." Sadly, industrial chemical pollution now begins in the *womb* and although the chemical industry claims that small amounts of toxic chemicals are not harmful, many experts dispute these claims.

In 2013, the American Congress of Obstetricians and Gynecologists and the American Society for Reproductive Medicine provided a powerful joint statement rejecting the chemical industry's claims of safety reassurance. The statement read: "Toxic chemicals in our environment harm our ability to reproduce, negatively affect pregnancies and are associated with numerous long-term health problems . . . . Toxic chemicals have long-lasting reproductive health effects . . . . prenatal exposure to certain chemicals is associated with stillbirth, miscarriage, birth defects, childhood cancers and impaired brain development in children."

Although many efforts are being made at the grassroots level to get this information out, it's still being largely ignored by federal and state lawmakers with the power to do something about it. So let's empower ourselves. Let's demand more transparency, and work together to find solutions. Let's open the door to our environment and examine some of our changed practices over the past few decades so we can see the full effect they're having on our children's health. Let's take a closer look at where some of the most dangerous toxins are coming from, the ways they're entering our children's bodies, and what precautionary steps we can take to reduce our children's exposure.

Section 2: The EPA's Role

I think the environment should be put in the category of our national security. Defense of our resources is just as important as defense abroad. Otherwise what is there to defend?
—Robert Redford

A YOUNG AGENCY (JOANNE)

After discovering what happened to so many children in Toms River, New Jersey, who were exposed to cancerous chemicals in their drinking water, I was angry and wanted someone to blame. These feelings intensified as I learned about the many uncontrolled toxic waste sites across the country identified by the EPA as Superfund sites. Why wasn't this governmental agency preventing these problems? I kept asking myself: How can these things happen? Why were toxic chemicals disposed of so irresponsibly? I soon realized just how young the EPA was, younger than me in fact. Many of the toxic dumping activities surrounding Superfund sites occurred decades ago—long before the EPA and laws pertaining to the environment even existed.

The EPA was established in 1970 to protect human health and the environment. Many important environmental laws were passed in the 1970s to help fulfill this mission, including the Clean Air Act, the Clean Water Act, and the Toxic Substances Control Act. Numerous safeguards were set up under these laws that improved the health of our environment and the health of our children. However, over the years these important laws have slowly been chipped away at by many different industries that didn't agree with the strict and sometimes costly regulations placed on their practices.

Much of this happened behind closed doors due to growing industry influence. Corporate giants spend billions of dollars influencing or lobbying Congress to vote for *their interests,* instead of what may be in the best interest of the American people or the environment. Industries have found ways to *weaken* original laws or obtain *exemptions* from them, making the EPA's job to protect us much harder. These and other loopholes have led to more venues for industrial toxic pollution and the widespread use of inadequately tested chemicals in many consumer products, changes that have compromised our environment and the health of our children.

As with our food, we face a problem with *transparency* in many aspects of the environment. We can't always see or smell a contaminant in our drinking water or a toxin in the air we breathe and the labels on consumer home products often fall short on content transparency as well. So there are no red flags to warn us of potential environmental dangers that can strongly influence our children's health.

Did You Know?

Some of the Health Effects of Chemicals May Include:

- Damage to our *immune* system, causing infections, allergies, and cancer
- Damage to our *endocrine* system, causing thyroid and adrenal disease or diabetes
- Damage to our *nervous* system, causing learning and behavior problems
- Damage to our *reproductive* system, causing changes and difficulty in reproductive health

---

Section 3: Unsafe Chemicals in Our Homes

Take care of the earth and she will take care of you.
—Author Unknown

THE CHEMICALLY SENSITIVE CHILD (CHRISTINE)

Before Kaleigh started on a full path to healing one of her worst allergic reactions as a toddler occurred on Christmas day. By late Christmas morning her face was so swollen she resembled a prize boxer. Her eyes were reduced to slits and any exposed skin was covered in hives. I was panicked, having no idea what she'd been exposed to that made her react so quickly. She hadn't eaten anything new recently. She hadn't had a chance to venture into anything poisonous because we were together all morning, as she sat under the Christmas tree playing with her new toys. What could cause her face to swell so severely?

Through the process of elimination and testing done over the next few days, we learned that her new plastic toy was the culprit. It contained several toxic chemicals Kaleigh was sensitive to, including formaldehyde. This event was long before warnings about toxic chemicals in plastic toys imported from China made the headlines. I wondered why a chemical like formaldehyde, classified as cancer-causing to humans, could ever be permitted in a toddler's toy. How many other consumer products also contain formaldehyde that she needed to be safeguarded from?

As an infant, Kaleigh also experienced a persistent, red, and dotted rash in her diaper area, which our doctor finally identified as a possible chemical reaction from exposure to antimony. How on earth was Kaleigh being exposed to antimony? Once again, through the process of elimination, the rash appeared to be from the disposable diapers. After we switched to all-natural diapers, the rash disappeared. I was shocked to find that even our disposable diapers can contain many harmful chemicals that can be either inhaled or absorbed into the skin and eventually make their way into the bloodstream. Disposable diapers can include chemicals like dioxins and sodium polyacrylate both linked to health problems including cancer, asthma, allergic reactions, and chemical burns.

For Kaleigh, it only takes veering off the all-natural path a little for her asthma and other immune problems to resurface. Each time she has a reaction it brings back the earlier years when I lived in constant fear, not knowing what each new day would bring with a child who could react quickly and severely to so many things. Having a chemically sensitive child taught me about the many dangers that lie hidden in our foods and household products. If a product was harmful, Kaleigh would undoubtedly react to it. This awareness also helped me safeguard my other children who were not chemically sensitive. Chemically sensitive children can be a blessing to us all because they bring into the light potential health problems from products we never would have suspected we needed protection from.

It seems only right that the chemical industry should have to clearly demonstrate that a substance is safe *before* it's used in children's products and other everyday products that fill our home. But because change will be *very slow* under the new TSCA reform, there will continue to be chemicals in a wide variety of children's products associated with health effects such as learning and behavioral problems, hormone disruption, and asthma. Whether it's flame retardants in car seats, triclosan in our soaps, or parabens in personal products, dangerous chemicals can enter our kids' bodies and negatively affect their health. Skin contact, inhalation, and ingestion through hand-to-mouth behaviors are ways our children are often exposed to toxic chemicals in our homes.

Did You Know?

 Personal care products (moisturizers, cleansers, cosmetics etc.) are not regulated under TSCA, instead these products are regulated by the FDA. Under our current law, the FDA does not assess the safety of these products. That job is left up to the product manufacturers themselves. Making matters worse, loopholes in our current laws allow many personal care products to end up on store shelves without all ingredients listed on product labels.

Because the products in our home surround our children every day, they may pose some of the greatest cumulative environmental health risks to our children. What follows is an overview of some chemical offenders that might be present in a nursery, courtesy of Toxic-Free Future (formerly known as Washington Toxics Coalition).

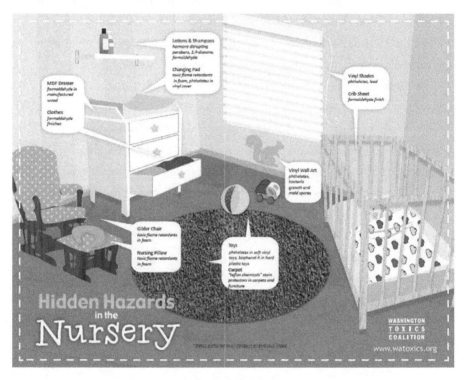

Graphic by Josh Schramm

Many of us can't imagine taking the time to go room by room identifying every possible toxic exposure to our children. But if you check out just the *one product* your child uses most and can swap it with a safer one, that's a start. This is one area where you can make an immediate difference. Every informed choice you make can help to improve the health and well-being of your family. At the end of this section, we've provided practical tools to help you quickly identify potential chemical hazards in your home so you can make safer choices.

It is important to stress that not all chemicals found in children's products are toxic and harmful, but some do put our children at *greater risk* than others. Below is a list of *chemicals of concern*, courtesy of Safer Chemicals, Healthy Families. These chemicals are important to focus on because they are linked to serious environmental and human health problems, including cancer and reproductive disorders. A few of them are discussed in more detail next. More background information on all of these chemicals, how to avoid them in products, and the important work of the Safer Chemicals, Healthy Families Coalition can be found in the Resource Guide (see Part 3 or at www.behindcloseddoorsthebook.com).

Did You Know?

Chemicals of Concern

Bisphenol A (BPA) * Formaldehyde * Heavy Metals (Mercury, Lead, Arsenic) * Hexane * Hexavalent Chromium * Methylene Chloride * Polychlorinated biphenyls (PCBs) and dichloro-diphenyl-trichloroethane (DDT) * Perfluorinated Compounds (Teflon and stain protectors) * Persistent, Bioaccumulative, and Toxic Chemicals (PBTs) * Phthalates * Toxic Flame Retardants (PBDEs, TDCP, and TCEP) * Tricholoroethylene (TCE) * Vinyl Chloride

---

Flame Retardants: A Lesson to Be Learned

Flame retardants seem to be everywhere and many of them are toxic. They can be found in our furniture, nursing pads, infant mattresses, car seats, clothing . . . the list goes on and on. But do we really need flame retardant chemicals linked to hormone disruption and cancer in our toddler's play tents and car seats? Because of the widespread use of flame retardant chemicals in the United States, Americans carry much higher levels of these chemicals in their bodies compared to others around the world. The good news is that most flame retardants hazardous to our children's health are now banned or being phased out. Although it appears we're working toward a solution, we do what we too often do: find a quick fix that substitutes one problem for another. A study by the Silent Spring Institute showed that many of the *replacement* flame retardants now being used instead of toxic polybrominated diphenyl ethers (PBDEs) still pose health hazards, including hormone disruption and cancer, while many others have unknown safety profiles. TDCP and TCEP are just two examples of replacement flame retardants that are *still* hazardous and *still* in use. We need to create safer products that provide *long-term* solutions for our children.

A Teachable Moment: Persistent Bioaccumlative Toxic Chemicals

The problem with figuring out that a chemical is extremely toxic and harmful after it's been in widespread use is that the damage is already done. Worse yet, is when the damaging effects have the ability to continue on long *after* a ban is imposed or we stop using it. This is especially true in the case of Persistent Bioaccumlative Toxic chemicals or PBTs. This class of chemicals doesn't break down easily, but instead hangs around and remains in our environment and our bodies for a long time after exposure (sometimes many years). Even when we try to trash a product containing a PBT, the hazardous substance persists in landfills and can be released into the air with the potential to travel long distances. PBT particles can then settle in our waterways and in our fish, and when we eat the fish, they settle in us.

Their persistence is why PBTs are so dangerous and why it's so important that we reform weak chemical laws. Some of our past mistakes with PBTs, like widespread use of the pesticide DDT, and our continued mistakes, like using brominated flame retardants in so many products, have initiated a cycle of harm. These toxic chemicals stay in both the environment and our bodies for a very long time because of their ability to accumulate or build up in an animal's fatty tissue or in our own human fatty tissue, like our breasts. Think breast cancer. Make the connection: PBTs are dangerous.

Some of the health effects of PBTs include DNA damage, cancer, neurological toxicity, brain toxicity, developmental toxicity, reproductive toxicity, and immune system damage. PBTs may be found in some of the following products: nonstick cookware, shampoo, cosmetics, stain-resistant carpets or anything containing brominated flame retardant materials. Many different chemicals (under different names) are considered PBTs.

For more information and a partial list of PBT chemical ingredients to avoid in products (courtesy of Safer Chemicals Healthy Families), see the Resource Guide. In the guide you can also find information on endocrine disruptors (some PBTs are also endocrine disruptors) and the "Dirty Dozen List" of endocrine-disrupting chemicals, courtesy of the EWG and the Keep A Breast Foundation.

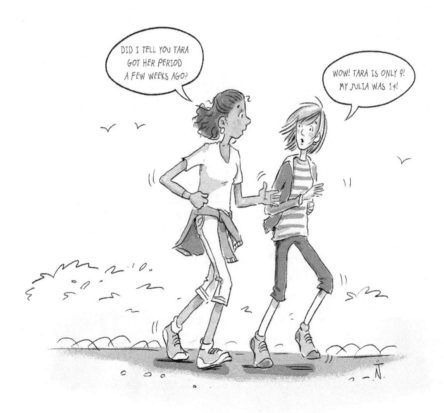

Plastics

Products containing plastic are everywhere. They are a big convenience for consumers, and often a big money saver for businesses, but the win-win ends there. A variety of potential health hazards, as well as huge environmental burdens, are associated with many plastic products in our homes, schools, and businesses. Because plastics are so pervasive in our environment, animals and marine life are also negatively affected, continuing the life cycle of dangerous chemicals in our food chain.

BPA is a well-known chemical of concern found in some plastics—but it's not our worst offender. According to the Center for Health, Environment, and Justice (CHEJ) the most toxic plastic affecting our children is *vinyl plastic*. Due to its widespread use in products commonly found in our schools (e.g., lunch boxes and binders) and homes (e.g., vinyl flooring) it is negatively impacting indoor air quality. As always, awareness is the first step. Safer alternatives to products made with vinyl plastic (and other dangerous plastics) are readily available to choose from.

The CHEJ says that polyvinyl chloride (PVC or vinyl) is a unique plastic material because it contains several dangerous chemical additives such as phthalates, lead, cadmium, and/or organotins that can all be toxic to children. During the PVC lifecycle, various toxic chemicals are released, which have been linked to developmental and learning disabilities, asthma, obesity, and cancer. Even *low levels* of exposure can be harmful to our children's bodies and may pose irreversible lifelong health threats. Be sure to avoid the recycling symbol with the **#3** on it or the initials PVC, which means that it was used in this product. See the Resource Guide for more information.

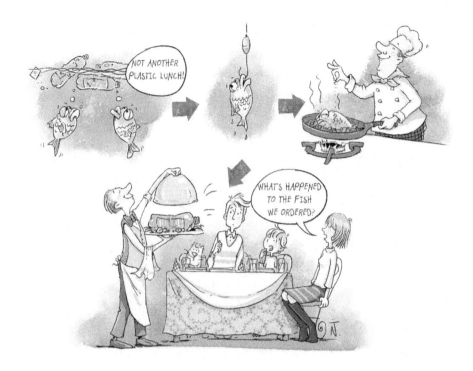

Practical Tools to Reduce Risks of Unsafe Chemicals in the Home

Below are some time-saving resources to help us identify the worst chemical offenders so we can reduce our family's exposures. More detailed information on the chemicals of concern listed earlier can be found in the Resource Guide (see Part 3 or www. behindcloseddoorsthebook.com).

✓ Check out all of the valuable resources and consumer tips provided by *Toxic-Free Future* (formerly known as Washington Toxics Coalition). They are a national leader in setting standards for toxic reforms in children's products. Their site includes many easy to follow tools to help you choose safer products and toys, as well as ways to create healthy home environments for your children. They also provide more detailed information on specific chemicals of concern, including how your children can be exposed to them, health concerns associated with that exposure, and ways to reduce exposure.

✓ Check out consumer product databases by the *Environmental Working Group* and the *Good Guide.* These sites provide information on both the personal products and home products your family uses most. Each site's database will give detailed health and safety information on thousands of home and personal care products. They also provide you with easy to understand safety ratings and allow you to conduct searches by the name of the product or by the individual chemical ingredients of a product.

✓ Check out *Safer Chemicals Safer Families Mind the Store Campaign,* which enlists consumers to use our buying power to influence retailers to remove toxic chemicals from products sold in stores. For example, through the efforts of this campaign, Lowe's committed to phasing out phthalates in all the flooring they sell by the end of 2015.

Did You Know?

 Of the 80,000+ chemicals in commercial use in the United States only about one-tenth of them has ever been assessed for potential human health effects. Under the *TSCA Reform* of 2016, the EPA is now charged with beginning to assess them. Change will be *slow*, as the EPA will only be required to have 20 of these chemicals under review at a time. Safety review for a chemical can take up to three years, and if the chemical fails the safety review, the EPA has another two years to finalize new restrictions on the chemical. (TSCA does not govern chemicals in food, cosmetics, or personal care products).

Section 4: Threats to Clean Air, Water, and Soil

> *Unless someone like you cares a whole awful lot,*
> *Nothing is going to get better. It's not.*
> —Dr. Seuss, *The Lorax*

Tens of thousands of chemicals are used by industries and businesses in the United States to make the things our society depends on: homes, electricity, food, clothing, automobiles, furniture, personal care products, electronics, and medicine. The EPA reports that American industries release over *four billion pounds of toxic chemicals* into our environment each year—into our soil, air, and water, the very resources our survival depends on. Many of these chemicals are known to increase the risk of cancers, developmental delays, reproductive problems, and a host of other health issues.

In addition to chemicals that are *known* to be toxic, industries also use and dispose of thousands of others whose potential risks to human health remain *unknown* due to inadequate testing. This is a primary reason why we need to continue to reform our chemical law (TSCA) and strengthen the EPA's power to protect us. Toxic releases are permitted because most federal or state regulators are trying to balance competing interests, such as the usefulness of plastic materials vs. the amount of toxins released during the lifecycle of these materials. The question becomes is it really in balance? Do public health considerations take a backseat to politics and industry profits? Is it possible that four billion pounds of toxic chemicals put into our environment each year could be contributing to our children's health problems?

Both the Clean Air Act and Clean Water Act allow the EPA to set standards of control for pollutants considered harmful to public health and the environment. These laws have resulted in huge victories for the health of our children, including reductions of lead and mercury in both our air and water. But despite these advances, air and water pollution remains a serious problem and more stringent standards are needed. Children are still at risk from breathing contaminants in air and drinking contaminants in water at levels that are significantly *below* the current EPA standards.

IN MY HOMETOWN (JOANNE)

I finally took some time to do research on the area where I grew up to see if any environmental concerns had been identified there. While on the EPA website, I quickly found that the Defense Department was the biggest owner of uncontrolled hazardous waste sites in the country, with 130 different military installations listed as Superfund sites. Both of the military sites near my childhood home were on the National Priority List (NPL) for Superfund sites and not far from the street I grew up on. The Navy Warfare Center (NAWC) in Warminster was identified as a hazardous waste site back in 1989, and the Willow Grove Naval Air Station Joint Reserve Base (NASJRB) in Horsham was named as a hazardous waste site in 1995. The EPA began investigating groundwater contamination at the NAWC in Warminster as early as 1979 and found heavy metals and many volatile organic compounds, including TCE and PCE, both associated with cancer in humans. Both sites are still being cleaned up or monitored by the EPA as a result of years of military operations using toxic chemicals, and other hazardous waste dating back to the 1950s or earlier.

Shortly after Patrick was diagnosed with a brain tumor, one of my childhood friends who grew up a few houses away from me learned that her three-year-old son also had a brain tumor. Within the last few years, another of my childhood friends who grew up directly across the street also had a small son diagnosed with a brain tumor. All the tumors were cancerous.

We now know that the effects of toxic chemicals can span generations. For example, harmful chemical exposures I experienced growing up could potentially have health effects on my children. In 2014, unregulated toxic chemicals were detected in both private drinking-water wells and municipal drinking-water wells in my childhood hometown and surrounding towns. There are no drinking-water standards for these chemicals, and samples were found at levels above the EPA's provisional health advisory levels.

Even more concerning is the type of chemicals that were detected in the drinking water. These persistent bioaccumulative chemicals (discussed earlier in this chapter) do not easily break down and can build up in the environment and the human body for years or decades. The specific chemicals found were PFOA (perfluorooctanoic acid) and PFOS (perfluorooctane sulfonate). PFOA and PFOS have a long half-life, which is the time it would take to expel half of a single dose from your body. According to the EPA, the half-life of both PFOA and PFOS is estimated at four years; eight years is a long time for a single dose of a toxic chemical to remain in your body.

The military sites near my home took responsibility for the PFOA and PFOS contamination. Both bases were using these toxic chemicals in routine firefighting exercises since the early 1970s and the levels detected in local drinking water samples were among some of the highest levels ever reported in our country.

Local water authorities had never been required to test for these unregulated chemicals until 2014 when an EPA program sampling for select unregulated chemicals in drinking water revealed their presence. Because public drinking water was never routinely tested for PFOA and PFOS, the EPA has no way to determine how long these chemicals have been affecting the residents' water supply. Both chemicals in question can cross the placenta during pregnancy and are linked to cancer and tumors in animals. They can also cause developmental, reproductive, and other adverse health effects. PFOS in particular has been shown to cause second-generation health effects in animal studies.

Everything I'd been uncovering crystallized, and I felt paralyzed by a stunning realization: I had spent my early pregnancy with Patrick in my hometown where these chemicals were detected.

I recalled what the doctor had told me years ago: "According to the report, Patrick's tumor sample showed that there was embryonic tissue in the very core indicating that its development may have started during pregnancy."

I felt sick as I read more about water contamination and the deep-rooted connection between health and the environment. According to the EPA community notice, "Continued exposure could increase body burden to levels that would result in adverse outcomes." What if we'd all been exposed to contaminated drinking water on a daily basis while growing up? What effect would this bioaccumulation of toxic chemicals have on a developing fetus? Could these chemicals have played a role in Patrick's brain tumor—and in the other cancers and chronic health problems reported by those living and working in the area during the past several decades? Was it a coincidence that three of us growing up together within the range of a few houses each had children of our own with brain tumors? Some of my childhood friends who later moved away also developed cancer or other serious health issues or had children with health problems—this important information will not be captured in current community health statistics or disease cluster investigations.

A part of me went into denial. It didn't want to know about all the conflicts of interest I was uncovering in the oversight of food, pharmaceuticals, and the environment. I'd just learned about decades of military cover-ups at Camp Lejeune in Jacksonville, North Carolina, where Marines and their families drank and bathed in contaminated water with toxins 240—3,400 times permitted by safety standards and linked to birth defects, many types of cancer, infertility, and a host of other medical problems. How many people who lived and worked in my hometown area could possibly have been exposed to toxic chemicals, radioactive materials, and other hazardous waste from military activities that entered our air, water, or soil? Although my questions will most likely go unanswered, I knew that I could not go back to my old life of childlike faith in our systems of protection.

Contamination and Quality Control of Our Water

Children are at higher risk from drinking-water contaminants because they consume more than *twice* the amount of water that adults do (based on their body weight percentage) and because water safety standards are based on an adult's safety not a child's.

The water supplied to our homes originates from various sources such as groundwater, streams, rivers, springs, or lakes in a watershed. Many of our local drinking-water sources unfortunately lack basic protections from everyday pollution (like metals, trash, and lawn fertilizer), as well as from toxic releases from industries, factory farms, or activities like fracking. These potential pollutants can all lead to drinking-water contamination with our tap water possibly containing things like arsenic, radon, lead, and pesticides.

Did You Know?

According to the Food and Water Watch the leading *health risk* of industrial toxic releases in water is *cancer.*

The EPA has established important water regulations in an effort to ensure that our drinking water is safe, including techniques to treat and disinfect drinking water. The EPA has also established legal *limits* on the levels of certain contaminants often found in our drinking water. For example, *arsenic* is the most common industrial toxic water pollutant posing risks to our drinking water. Because arsenic has a maximum contaminant level (MCL) set by the EPA, the water treatment facilities in our various communities must test for arsenic. If arsenic is detected at levels above the MCL, a treatment plan is implemented before it enters our drinking water. Arsenic levels must also be reported to the EPA.

But here's the problem. There are so many different chemicals and other contaminants being used and released into groundwater these days—many of them suspected or known to pose health hazards—that the EPA is having a hard time establishing MCLs for all of them (especially when industries try to block these efforts). According to a report by the Food and Water Watch, there are *hundreds* of different *toxic* chemicals being released into our drinking-water sources—and only seventy-seven chemicals have a MCL set by the EPA. If no MCL is set for a toxic chemical, there is *no required testing*. Local drinking-water treatment plants *do not* have to *test* or *remediate* for hundreds of chemicals known to be toxic, including many known to cause cancer, and for thousands of other potentially toxic chemicals.

As a consequence, many different chemicals like *perchlorate* (used in rocket fuel, flares, etc.) and *triclosan* (antimicrobial pesticide found in soaps, body lotions, and toothpaste), which may cause adverse health effects in our children, can currently *find their way* into our drinking water. So too can some of the toxic chemicals used in fracking operations or identified at a local EPA Superfund site. When you read the water quality report that comes in the mail from your local public water supplier, it's important to understand that the water quality test results aren't the *whole picture* of what you're drinking every day.

- ✓ The results only reflect contaminants *that have been tested*.
- ✓ They only contain *average* levels for most contaminants, as opposed to all test results.
- ✓ They are not required to disclose many *unregulated* chemicals they *may* have tested for.
- ✓ They are not required to disclose chemicals found above *health guidelines*—only MCL violations are required to be reported, and MCL limits are often *much higher* than government *health* guidelines.

So when your water quality report is glowing, just realize that it doesn't *necessarily* mean that your water is free from contaminants or toxins posing health risks to your children. But the good news is that there are definitely more things we can do to identify and control the contaminants in our drinking water, as compared to something like our outdoor air.

However, the answer is *not as simple as bottled water*. Contrary to popular belief, bottled water has proven to be *no safer* than tap water and often comes from the same sources as tap water. Bottled water also creates more pollution, further harming our environment. Plastic bottles can also leach the hormone disrupting chemical BPA.

Summary

 The EPA has established important water regulations in an effort to ensure that our drinking water is safe, including techniques to treat and disinfect drinking water. However, due to the sheer volume of potential contaminants that could end up in our water, it's possible for hundreds of chemicals known to be toxic to go undetected at our local water treatment facilities.

Practical Tools: Protecting Our Children's Drinking Water

The best solution we've found to protect our children's drinking water is to find out what contaminants are being released into our communities and what contaminants are present in our drinking water, and then purchase a good water filtration system that filters specifically for those contaminants. You can find an easy step-by-step process to follow in the Resource Guide (see in Part 3 or www. behindcloseddoorsthebook.com). By simply entering your zip code on an EPA website, you can effortlessly find out what industrial toxins are being released into the neighborhood where you live. You can also quickly view the water quality (and air quality) where you live. See the Resource Guide for more detailed information on these community resources.

Section 5: Environmental Practices of Concern

When one tugs at a single thing in nature,
he finds it attached to the rest of the world.
—John Muir

In this section we will share a few of our country's changed environmental practices over the past few decades that are increasing toxic pollution in our environment and impacting human health. These and many other environmental practices need to be examined more closely so we can improve the well-being of our children. The more of us that awaken to just how toxic many of our practices are the greater chance we have to change them.

Sewage Sludge: Recycling of Human Waste

Wastewater treatment plants are designed to remove various pathogens, metals, and toxic chemicals from wastewater. The removed materials left over from this process concentrate into a semisolid substance referred to as sewage sludge. Over eight million tons of sewage sludge are used or disposed of each year in the United States. In the past, local governments could legally dispose of sewage sludge in three ways: landfills, incinerators, or by discharging them into waterways using permits. Since 1992, due to the Ocean Dumping Reform Act, the waste management industry has needed to find a new place to dump sewage sludge that had previously been dumped into U.S. waterways. You will never guess where much of it *eventually* ended up—U.S. farmland.

In 1993, many municipalities found that the cheapest option for disposing of this hazardous waste was to partake in the government program of "recycling" sewage sludge to farmers as fertilizer for food crops. In order for sewage sludge to be eligible for land application it must first undergo a strict chemical, thermal, or biological treatment process. The treated sewage sludge (also known as "biosolids") contains beneficial nutrients useful as a fertilizer. However, in addition to nutrients it may also contain heavy metals, toxicants, and pathogens.

Think about that. What we put down our sinks, drains, or toilets can eventually make its way into sludge, then be processed or "cleaned," and then sprayed on food crops. According to the Center for Food Safety, "(W)hile certain sanitation processes do decrease some health risks, chemicals such as PCBs, flame retardants, heavy metals, and endocrine disrupters—many of which are carcinogens—are not filtered out. Instead, they accumulate in the soil and are taken up by crops, putting human health at risk."

Is it any coincidence that foodborne illnesses have increased more than 700 percent since this practice began in the early 1990s? Serious illnesses in humans and livestock as well as adverse environmental impacts have been linked to land application of sewage sludge. The EPA only monitors nine of the thousands of pathogens commonly found in sewage sludge, putting our children and our environment at risk. This program and its regulations have been criticized by many consumer and environmental advocacy groups, as well as the CDC. Studies have shown that many pharmaceuticals regularly excreted into sewage waste are now finding their way into food crops through sewage sludge—including chemotherapy and antipsychotic drugs. How can this newer practice not have health effects on our children? This is another reason to "Go Organic" since the USDA organic certification prohibits the use of sewage sludge on organic farmland.

TOO CLOSE FOR COMFORT (JOANNE)

When Patrick was two years old, my husband was transferred for work, and we moved just a few miles north of a Pennsylvania nuclear power plant. Every time I drove by the two reactors and saw the huge plume of smoke rising into the sky, I got an uneasy feeling in my stomach. I passed them twice a day as I traveled to and from coaching a high school field hockey team. At the time I was pregnant with Colin, and Patrick was just a toddler, usually fast asleep in his car seat. Within a year of our moving there, our son Colin was born, eight weeks prematurely. Our next-door neighbor worked at the nuclear reactor and I often drilled him with questions. He constantly reassured me that the plant was perfectly safe and no radiation was ever released. Although I'm sure he was saying what he believed to be true, my gut kept telling me something different. Twenty years later, I realize that my initial instincts were probably right.

Nuclear Power Plants

There's growing concern about increased cancer rates in children living in areas surrounding nuclear power plants in the United States. Similar concerns were a major factor in Germany's recent decision to phase out all such plants in their country. Children are among the most vulnerable to (and least protected from) radiation exposure. Radiation exposure can damage cells and cause birth defects, immune and endocrine disorders, and radiation-induced cancer. In 2006, the National Academies of Science issued a definitive report on radiation exposure, concluding that even *low levels* of radiation can cause human health problems. Additionally, the current "acceptable" exposure standards in the United States are based on the "standard man" and do not take into account the more serious effects of radiation exposure on children, pregnant women, and their unborn babies.

Nuclear power plants generate approximately 18 percent of our country's electricity. Although they produce electricity with less carbon emissions than other fossil fuels, such as coal, it's far from *clean* energy, due to the large amounts of radioactive waste left behind. It's also far from *safe* energy due to the radioactive materials it releases into the environment during everyday operations along with its vulnerability to accidents or a terrorist attack.

Contrary to what many believe, a nuclear power plant doesn't have to melt down to release radioactive materials into the environment. Radioactive materials are released in low doses daily and federal regulations permit them. You can't see, smell, feel, or taste these emissions and there's no technology that can filter out all the radioactive liquids, gases, and particles released by a typical reactor. They end up in our air, water, and soil, potentially affecting food and water sources along with our children's health.

When we looked into the practices at a local nuclear reactor these facts were reaffirmed. For instance, radioactive materials have indeed been detected in the surrounding community's sediment, air, water, and even cow's milk. These are the same radioactive materials used to operate the reactors. The billion-dollar corporation that owns the reactor receives exemptions to federal water laws including a *water pollution permit* allowing them to discharge (via monitored pathways) dangerous toxins and radionuclides into the Schuylkill River, a drinking-water source for almost two million people in the Philadelphia area.

Studies have shown that after some nuclear power plants began operations, local communities saw increases in cancer rates and other illnesses. For instance, the nuclear power plant noted above opened in 1985, and health statistics for the communities in closest proximity to the reactors include childhood cancer rates rising to 92.5 percent higher than the national average by the late 1990s. Infant mortality rates were also much higher for communities near the power plant than for the closest major cities and the state average. Despite these numbers, those working in the nuclear power industry continually deny any correlation. One particular study conducted in this same community, a children's baby tooth study, is hard to refute. Baby teeth are an undeniable way to prove children's exposure to certain radioactive materials because one type of radionuclide (Strontium 90) routinely released from nuclear power plants settles in bones. Teeth are similar to bones and baby teeth can absorb this dangerous radionuclide if a child is exposed.

Area residents near this nuclear power plant with higher than normal incidence of childhood cancer rates were asked to donate their children's baby teeth, after they fell out. The results showed the presence of Strontium 90 in the baby teeth of area residents at some of the highest levels ever found in the United States. How can an industry continually turn a blind eye to the potential adverse health effects of their practices? How can they say it's a "safe" or "permissible" background level of radiation exposure for communities surrounding nuclear power plants, when a 2006 radiation report (BIER) concluded that there is "no safe level" of exposure? Local residents deserve the whole truth. Electricity generation from nuclear power plants involves the release of radioactive materials, which remain pervasive in the environment for days, weeks, years, and even decades (due to long half-life) and can damage human health. According to the Union of Concerned Scientists, the Nuclear Regulatory Commission, who is charged with oversight of the nuclear power industry, has repeatedly violated its monitoring responsibilities to the public, citing hundreds of case summary reports where unmonitored, uncontrolled, or uncapped leaks and spills took place at individual nuclear power plants.

Germany has already made the smart and ethical decision to end their reliance on nuclear power, citing one reason as the increased cancer risks to children living nearby. Instead, our politicians (who often receive industry contributions) support laws that provide subsidies and toxic release permits full of exemptions to the nuclear industry. We can do better than this for our children.

Power plants are also responsible for 50 to 60 percent of the toxic pollutants discharged into our surface waters each year, contributing to the degradation of many of our nation's drinking-water sources and putting human health at risk.

Power plant wastewater contains heavy metals and other toxins associated with birth defects, cancer, and other health problems.

*[Authors' note: The EPA recommends the use of a **reverse osmosis water filtration system** to reduce radiation exposure from household drinking water. It can remove up to 99 percent of radionuclides, as well as many other water contaminants, including disease-causing contaminants, metals, arsenic, asbestos, and additional chemical contaminants.]*

Roundup: Much More than Green Lawns and Green Veggies

Since the 1970s many of us have been using weed killers like Roundup (an herbicide) on our lawns and in our landscaping without much thought to its effect on the environment or our health. As discussed in the food chapter, *glyphosate*, the key ingredient in Roundup, is heavily used in industrialized farming and has increased sharply since the development of GMO food crops in the early 1990s. This toxic substance doesn't just go away after it's been sprayed, but ends up on our lawns, in our soil, in our water, and on our food crops. Its potential to negatively affect our health is only beginning to be understood.

An MIT study published in the peer-reviewed April 2013 edition of *Entropy* suggests that glyphosate may prove to be the most biologically disruptive chemical in our environment, causing chronic, long-term health problems, especially for our children. Glyphosate may explain a large number of the recent increases in chronic diseases and conditions experienced by both children and adults, including inflammatory bowel disease, obesity, depression, ADHD, autism, cancer, infertility, and developmental malformations. According to the authors of the study, the chemicals' negative impact on the human body is "insidious and manifests slowly over time, as inflammation damages cellular systems throughout the body."

This study didn't make headline news, but what did make news a few weeks after it was published was that the EPA *raised* the limits for how much glyphosate is allowed on our children's fruits and vegetables. The USDA also continues to approve additional new glyphosate-resistant GMO crops with the potential to add more glyphosate to our food, our environment, and ultimately our children's bodies.

In early 2015, the World Health Organization (WHO) classified glyphosate as a probable carcinogen to humans and the WHO's concerns were not just limited to exposure to *high* doses of glyphosate. Studies have shown that *very low levels* of glyphosate can mimic the hormone estrogen and stimulate the growth of breast cancer cells, even at doses far *below* those allowed in U.S. drinking water. A recent pilot study conducted by Sustainable Pulse and Mom's Across America showed that glyphosate was also detected in the breast milk of mothers. All of the scientific information available on glyphosate supports our maternal instincts that its widespread use in the home, in industrial products, and on GMO food crops is a contributing factor to many rising health problems in our country.

Fracking

Hydraulic fracturing (fracking) is a relatively new process of natural gas and oil extraction from the Marcellus shale running underground in many states across the country. Although this controversial technology has led to the rapid increase in oil and gas production in the United States, it appears to be in need of more regulations without convenient loopholes that protect the industry at the expense of both human health and the health of the environment. For instance, the industry enjoys certain exemptions under the Safe Drinking Water Act, the Clean Air Act, and the Clean Water Act, and from reporting any of their toxic releases to the EPA's Toxic Release Inventory Program. Since fracking sites can be located within a few hundred feet of our homes and schools, the practice may threaten the water our children drink and the air our children breathe.

Fracking is different from traditional gas and oil extraction. Millions of gallons of water and thousands of gallons of toxic chemicals are mixed with sand to create fracking fluid. The fluid is then pumped into the wells at high pressure to create cracks in the shale so gas or oil can then flow back up through the well for use. During this process methane gas and toxic chemicals can potentially leach out from the system and contaminate groundwater or air. Up to 600 chemicals are used in fracking fluid, including those known to cause cancer: mercury, lead, uranium, ethylene glycol, hydrochloric acid, and formaldehyde. Due to confidentiality rights of the industry (similar to GMOs) many of the chemicals used are not required under federal law to be shared with local residents living nearby (although many consumer advocacy groups are working to change this). Why does the industry stand protected and not the health and well-being of the community?

Drinking-water contamination is among the top concerns of many residents of fracking communities. During the fracking process it is possible for well water and groundwater to be contaminated with toxic chemicals, methane gas, and sometimes radioactive materials. If contamination does take place, these same chemicals, gases, and radioactive materials can end up in the drinking water of nearby cities and towns. There have been thousands of health complaints filed in the United States by those living near fracking operations reporting sensory, respiratory, and neurological damage in humans. In Pennsylvania alone, we've seen more than a dozen incidents where public water treatment facilities have accepted natural gas wastewater, treated it improperly, and discharged the toxins back into source waters used for drinking water. Under current federal drinking-water standards, wastewater treatment plants do not test for all toxins used in fracking or remediate for all of them.

The natural gas and oil companies involved in fracking who reap billions in profits enjoy financial subsides and many exemptions from reporting their toxic releases under several different laws. Should they be exempt from accountability? Are the exemptions related to the fact that the industry pumped nearly 240 million dollars into our lawmakers' political campaigns since 1990, not to mention what they spend on lobbying efforts? The fracking industry goes largely unregulated while the local residents in fracking communities are left to deal with any lasting repercussions of the practice.

What will this do to our home state of Pennsylvania, where Marcellus shale runs under two-thirds of the ground and laws permit gas and oil drilling to take place in any municipality across the state? How will this affect our water, our food crops, and other agriculture that Pennsylvania is so dependent on? What will this do to the health of children living nearby fracking operations? A 2015 health study titled "Health Hazards to Fetuses, Infants, and Young Children in Heavily Fracked Areas of Pennsylvania," found that heavily fracked counties have 13.9 percent greater infant mortality, 23.6 percent greater perinatal mortality, 12.4 percent more premature births, and 35.1 percent more cancer in children ages zero to four when compared to counties without fracking. When will we learn cause and effect of our practices?

According to the Union of Concerned Scientists, "The fast-paced growth of this practice is driving many landowners and communities to make decisions without fully investigating the practice and potential impacts on local air and water quality, community health, safety, the economy, the environment, and overall quality of life." Yes, we need energy and we need to become less dependent on foreign countries for our energy needs. But until we can be assured that the health of our children and the environment is not being compromised, fracking cannot be the best answer.

LOCAL LIMITS (CHRISTINE)

Around Labor Day 2015 I was notified of a local township meeting scheduled to address fracking in my community. I'd attended the past three meetings and was hopeful that we could find a way to stop this from happening in our town. Due to the late notice, many declined the meeting invitation, which left me frustrated. Many were still unaware of the potential health effects to our children and the environment. An hour before the meeting, I called Joanne and expressed my frustration over the late notice of the meeting keeping many from attending.

"You can't control that," Joanne had said. "Don't give up now. Forget about who's not there and be thankful for those that are. That's what you build on."

At the meeting, we learned that our township leaders were trying to enact an ordinance designating a drilling location for fracking in our town that would be least harmful to our community. Due to state law in Pennsylvania, without this ordinance in place, the energy industry could come into our town and pick any spot they wanted for fracking—next to a school or day care or hospital. Most people don't realize that most often local governments remain essentially powerless to stop fracking operations in their community.

A neighboring community was also trying to keep a natural gas pipeline from being built that would move natural gas fracked from

Marcellus shale in northern Pennsylvania to markets in southern Pennsylvania and New Jersey. This proposed pipeline was less than ten miles from my house. Once again, municipalities in Pennsylvania only hold the power to possibly change the route but are unlikely to stop a pipeline project.

As I sat at my local township meeting, I learned about some newly published statistics on the health effects on children in heavily fracked areas that included, among other things, a considerably increased risk for cancer. As I listened I was afraid for those families and my own, especially Kaleigh, with her autoimmune issues and chemical sensitivities. The children represented in these statistics could be my children or anyone else's children. I thought to myself, "What kind of a society allows business interests to take priority over the health of its children?"

Did You Know?

 A 2012 study out of Cornell's College of Veterinary Medicine published in *New Solutions: A Journal of Environmental and Occupational Health Policy*, suggests that hydraulic fracturing may be sickening and killing our pets, farm animals, fish, and other wildlife, as well as humans. The study looked at cases in Colorado, Louisiana, New York, Ohio, Pennsylvania, and Texas. It included reports of sick animals, stunted growth, and dead animals after exposure to hydraulic fracturing spills from dumping of the fluid into streams and from workers slitting the lining of a wastewater impoundment (evaporation ponds) so that it would drain and be able to accept more waste. Researchers said that it was hard to assess health impacts because of industry lobbying that greatly influenced legislation allowing companies to keep proprietary chemicals used in the fracking process secret. These laws remain barriers to making direct links to illness and death and helps protect industry from being held legally responsible for any contamination.

Section 6: Encouraging News and Practical Tools for Change

> *We shall require a substantial new manner*
> *of thinking if mankind is to survive.*
> —Albert Einstein

WHOSE BACKYARD? (CHRISTINE)

In the fall of 2015, as Joanne and I were finishing this book, I became aware of another serious environmental threat to a neighboring community. A local environmental activist, asked me if I'd rally as many residents as possible to attend a Pennsylvania Department of Environmental Protection (DEP) public hearing to stop a hazardous waste treatment facility from being built about eleven miles from my home. The plans involved annually treating 210,000 tons of raw wastewater, holding toxins such as mercury, cadmium, and lead. The incineration part of this process would produce more than 30 tons of air pollution a year. I grew even more concerned when I learned the proposed site would be one of the largest medical waste facilities in our country, processing highly toxic pharmaceutical waste only half a mile from the Delaware River, a source of drinking water for millions of people. It is also located in close proximity to a farm and community sports fields. I was alarmed by the facility's potential effects on air quality for those living nearby, especially for children like Kaleigh who may have asthma. When I attended the DEP meeting, I was further disturbed to learn that the company proposing the facility had a poor track record, with numerous environmental violations.

The Philadelphia Water Authority also submitted comments on the application for the proposed facility, bringing attention to the hazardous materials that would be transported via regional waterways and the significant risk it posed to the drinking-water supply of millions of people. Most disheartening was that according to a local Clean Air

Council, the air quality in the community was already poor due to an existing waste incinerator already in operation that sits adjacent to the proposed site, exposing low-income and minority populations to toxic air pollution.

Community Action for Environmental Justice

Where we live can be a strong and often overlooked influence on the health of our children. Unfortunately, many of us can't control where we live and families of low income often carry the brunt of many environmental threats to our health. Lower-income neighborhoods are often targeted to host facilities with some of the highest levels of toxic industrial releases in our country, such as power plants, chemical factories, and landfills. Those who live, work, and play closest to the sources of pollution often suffer great health disparities, including higher rates of cancer, birth defects, developmental delays, and infertility. Environmental justice is a basic right we all deserve. Conversations like "Not in my backyard" need to become "Not in anyone's backyard." When we change our thinking, we can begin to ensure health and safety for *all* children.

Over the past two years, we've both been drawn into grassroots activism in the hope of improving the health of our own local communities. Here are a few encouraging examples of ways many communities are pushing back against environmental threats, highlighting the power we hold when we join together for a common cause.

Communities Standing Up for Environmental Justice

✓ Over the past several years, more than a hundred small towns in New York have organized grassroots efforts that successfully enacted local bans or moratoriums on fracking operations and other gas drilling in their communities. Finally, in December 2014 the entire state of New York banned fracking due to public health concerns regarding the practice. These victories are helping to protect the health of New York residents and the environment itself.

✓ At the time a large chemical company announced plans to build a new polyvinyl chloride (PVC) plant near Convent, Louisiana, the town had roughly two thousand people. Eighty percent of the residents were black and 43 percent poor. Convent already carried the burden of four large polluting factories and was located in a county known as "cancer alley." Residents fought back, organizing themselves and gaining the support of various political, educational, and religious organizations. Within two years this small community successfully stopped the PVC plant from setting up in their town.

✓ Beyond Toxics is a small grassroots environmental health organization in Eugene, Oregon. It took action when an assistant teacher in West Eugene alerted members that children were having trouble breathing during recess due to the ammonia and creosote fumes from a nearby factory. Beyond Toxics got the EPA to investigate the polluting factory, which revealed many lax air-quality controls. The event sparked them to begin an *environmental justice project* in this area with high levels of toxic industrial pollution, which is also home to higher proportions of low income and Latino families. The project established a correlation between toxic air pollution in their community and increased asthma rates in local children, which were 77 percent higher than for school children in surrounding districts. Beyond Toxics is working to hold local industries accountable for their air pollution and to improve the health of their community.

Green Chemistry

We mentioned earlier that U.S. industries admit to releasing four billion pounds of toxic chemicals each year; the EPA has said that these releases are "inevitable." We disagree—somewhat. Although some releases may be inevitable, many toxic chemicals can now be replaced with technology called Green Chemistry. This is where toxic substances are reduced or eliminated in products to protect the health of humans and the environment. Many companies are turning to this technology to make their consumer products safer for our children and the environment. Johnson and Johnson is one example of a company that made this commitment to safer products. This change will have far-reaching positive effects, because Johnson and Johnson is also the maker of brands such as Neutrogena,

Aveeno, Clean and Clear, RoC, and Lubriderm. Please know that there are many ways companies can reduce toxicity in our consumer products and the resulting industrial releases into our air, water, and soil. Imagine living in a country where stricter chemical regulations dictated that all companies used green chemistry to ensure the health and well-being of our children.

Green Energy

Everything we learned about nuclear power and fracking made us realize the importance of clean, sustainable energy sources, like solar and wind. Green energy is *already available* and, as consumer demand increases, it is slowly becoming just as affordable as other sources. According to the Union of Concerned Scientists, renewable energy resources generate electricity with little or no pollution or global warming emissions and could reliably provide up to 40 percent of U.S. electricity needs by 2030 and 80 percent by 2050. You can support the clean energy industry by signing up for renewable energy for your home. More and more electricity customers now have an option of purchasing "green power" from clean energy sources.

Your electricity can come from the same provider through the same lines completely uninterrupted; but it will only pull from clean, renewable sources such as solar and wind instead of from coal, gas and oil fracking, or other potentially harmful sources like nuclear power. Contact your electricity provider for more information on how your electricity bill can support the clean energy industry.

Environmental Laws and Political Solutions

Some of us might not be aware of how widespread our children's exposure to toxic chemicals and other environmental contaminants has become over the past few decades. Even more importantly, we may not have realized the critical role the environment actually plays in our children's health. As mothers we can certainly make different choices in our daily lives to help reduce risks for our children, but to create real solutions we need to do something together on a much larger scale.

Politics and laws are truly our lifeline because they drive consumer protection and safety. Laws govern much of what industries can and cannot do. So, if we want to change the way things are, our voice in politics is of great importance. Look at our current environmental practices—the reality is that big money from industries strongly influences our legislation. As individuals this problem seems overwhelming, but if we join together in a concerted effort this is a grassroots battle we can win. We'll talk more about politics and working together for change in Chapter 9.

TREVOR'S LAW (JOANNE)

Throughout the United States, there are geographic areas known as "disease clusters" with unexpected and unusually high incidence of birth defects, cancer, and other diseases in children and adults. For example, the town of Toms River, New Jersey, proved to be a childhood cancer cluster after chemical companies treated the town as a private dumping ground for decades. Unfortunately, proving a true cause and effect relationship between environmental contaminants and a disease is something that takes a lot of effort, time, and money.

I remember wondering about many of these same things when Patrick was initially diagnosed with a cancerous brain tumor because a few other children from our small town also had brain tumors at the same time. Was this a coincidence? Was this environmental? Could it have stemmed from the nuclear power plant fifteen miles away? Was it from our community's Superfund site that hadn't been remediated yet?

All of the questions that ran through my mind are often the ones that get explored when looking into disease clusters in a community. However, in reality, when parents see patterns and raise concern for several sick children in the neighborhood, there are no real resources to assist us in a coordinated effort to investigate potential common factors or related causes. Luckily, thanks to new legislation passed with TSCA REFORM in 2016, this may soon change.

About two years ago, I was introduced to a woman by the name of Charlie Smith. Her son, Trevor, was diagnosed with the same type of brain tumor as Patrick. Charlie and I were both concerned about environmental contaminants and the potential role they played in our children's brain tumors. She had gotten involved in political activism while Trevor was in cancer treatments. During that time, she learned about industrial toxic dumping and cover-ups in their small Idaho town, events that contaminated both the lake her son swam in and the town's drinking water. Their town of 1,700 had a seemingly higher number of brain cancers, but when it was brought to the attention of government agencies, the Smiths were told that their community was too small to warrant an investigation into a cancer cluster. She fought back and helped inspire bipartisan legislation known as "Trevor's Law." It was signed into law in 2016 as an addendum to the TSCA Reform.

The law provides protection to communities suspecting a disease cluster by allocating resources to help determine whether there is a connection between "clusters" of cancer—and contaminants in the surrounding environment.

Charlie explained how this legislation would ensure that government agencies coordinated their efforts and worked with experts at academic institutions to investigate potential disease clusters and provide meaningful assistance to communities. I was so excited to hear that this was passed and thanked her for all her efforts. This law would help so many people, including those in my childhood hometown, as residents past and present were very concerned about the high number of people affected with cancer and other illnesses possibly associated with two decades of activity from a pair of local military operations on the National Priority List for EPA Superfund sites.

After hanging up, I realized that Charlie had buttressed everything I'd been learning through my own research. She shared my same frustration about environmental loopholes allowing industrial toxic pollution and gaps in our systems of protection. She also validated to me the importance of transparency surrounding the health effects of environmental contaminants. Identifying any problem empowers us to choose a course of action to begin to do something about it.

Environmental Medicine

There is help available for many who suffer from the environmental health effects we discussed in this chapter—help some of us may be unaware of— because it comes from an emerging field known as environmental medicine. Environmental medicine, which we touched on in the food chapter, recognizes that there are *causes* for all illnesses—and that causes *may* include what we are exposed to in our environment such as air, food, and water contaminants, radiation, and toxic chemicals. By acknowledging the simple concept of *cause and effect* in our health, the focus of environmental medicine is on the *prevention* of an illness instead of waiting for an illness to emerge and then *reacting* to it.

More and more mothers are turning to environmental medicine, and the many medical doctors (MDs) who practice it, because it *sometimes* provides answers to our children's health issues when traditional medicine comes up short. Environmental medicine can be the difference between identifying and treating the root cause of an illness vs. simply managing symptoms for years. Doctors practicing environmental medicine and other integrative medical practices may prescribe medication, such as a steroid cream for short-term relief of a skin rash or an antibiotic for a recurring infection. But they know that treatment entails much more than controlling the associated symptoms. They're more focused on finding the source of the problem and then working to restore the body's natural balance, avoiding the long-term use of medication whenever possible. This balanced approach to medicine can offer help to many of today's children suffering from illnesses related to environmental health effects.

For example, most mothers would never make the connection between their baby's asthma and disposable diapers. Yet some diapers can contain harmful chemicals that can cause or exacerbate asthma; peer-reviewed medical journal articles are dedicated to this very topic. Certain chemicals or foods can also be a trigger for asthma, allergies, and children's behavioral problems. Environmental medicine does not hold the solution for *every* child, but it's worth exploring when dealing with a chronic health issue. We have both used environmental medicine practices and seen amazing improvements in our children's health and our own.

It's widely acknowledged that the environment may contribute to a variety of diseases or health disorders, including autism. In the next chapter we share a powerful story about a little girl diagnosed with autism at age three. This story speaks volumes about the benefits of integrating environmental medicine into the overall healthcare of your child. Information on how to locate a physician practicing environmental medicine in your area and a list of different environmental health and environmental medicine organizations and their varying missions and philosophies can be found in the Resource Guide (see Part 3 or www.behindcloseddoorsthebook.com).

Chapter 8

AN AUTISM STORY OF HOPE

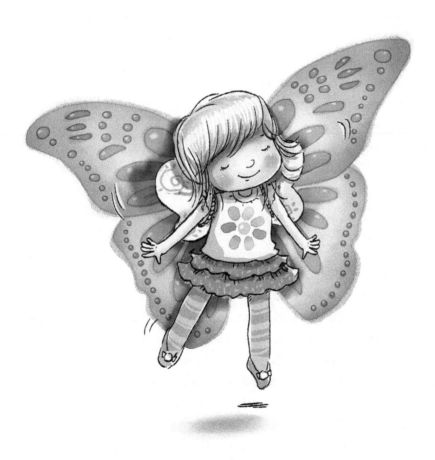

The significant problems we face cannot be solved
by the same level of thinking that created them.
—Albert Einstein

t's unfortunate that traditional medicine has been unable to provide children diagnosed with autism any real hope for a cure. Early intervention programs provide much needed assistance in managing this illness, but there's no magic pill for autism and all of its associated symptoms. Many resilient parents have set out on journeys to find their own solutions that often include specialty fields, such as environmental medicine and the use of complementary and integrative therapies.

We believe that autistic children, growing in numbers every day, are becoming our greatest teachers, serving as special messengers for our generation. What they and their families have endured, uncovered, and shared with the rest of us may prove to be one of the most valuable lessons we need to learn at this time in history. Like the canaries sent into the coal mines to help detect and warn of chemical dangers inside, these highly sensitive children are now opening our eyes to the toxins that lie hidden in many of our current practices. Many autistic children seem to be more susceptible to the harmful effects of chemicals, heavy metals, and other contaminants found in the environment, in foods, in consumer products, and even in some medical protocols.

The message here is simple: when harmful exposures are eliminated, many autistic children experience improvements in symptoms. These pioneering children and their parents are gifts to the world, teaching us about the important need for change. A mother's love is a powerful and protective force. So too is knowledge. With these two forces, a mother can even usher in miracles. Against the odds, my (Joanne's) niece, Kate, overcame a diagnosis of autism. Her success story would not have been possible without the sheer perseverance of her mother, Mary, who never stopped learning and looking for answers. Their story touches every topic we have covered in this book and bears witness to how real these threats are to our children's health. Although we can only provide a condensed version here, we hope it gives a face to all of the childhood statistics we've presented, and provides a glimpse into the daily struggles and small victories associated with a chronic illness.

THE ROAD LESS TRAVELED (MARY)

My daughter Kate was diagnosed with autism at age three. Like most mothers, I was devastated and shocked at the diagnosis. At the time, Kate seemed in many ways intellectually advanced compared to some of her peers; she completed complicated puzzles and patterns quickly and had an almost photographic memory. However, socially and behaviorally, she exhibited some telltale symptoms of autism that were hard to acknowledge. Kate's diagnosis was when the real challenge of parenthood began for us, and we set out on a long and difficult journey of self-education and seeking answers that continues today.

Our beautiful daughter is now twelve and no longer has the label of autism. This is reason to celebrate, and why I want to share all I've learned with you so that others may also benefit. This is all about giving each other hope. As mothers we have the power to make a difference in our children's lives. For me, it started with every educated and conscious choice I made for Kate.

After she was first diagnosed, we soon got her into various early intervention therapies, including physical therapy, speech therapy, occupational therapy, music therapy, and DIR/Floortime (play) therapy. All were recommended by the neurodevelopmental pediatrician (NDP) who gave us the diagnosis. This was an intense effort that consumed our lives for the next several years.

As difficult as it was to accept this diagnosis, I found it much harder to accept that these traditional therapies could only lead to **some** improvements in Kate's ability to function, without offering the hope of ever overcoming her diagnosis. There had to be more we could provide, and if it was out there I was determined to find it.

Luckily, I had a dear friend whose son also had autism. Since my friend was several years ahead of me on her journey, she essentially became my "autism mentor" and strongly encouraged me to make an appointment with a physician who specialized in environmental medicine. She knew firsthand that this doctor would immediately offer us additional solutions beyond what was recommended by the NDP. She was right. Significant blood, urine, and stool testing ordered by the environmental doctor confirmed food sensitivities that included dairy, gluten, corn, and bananas. Kate had an obscure condition shared by many autistic children, known as leaky gut syndrome. Tests also identified numerous vitamin and mineral deficiencies present in her body. We started her on a regimen of supplements to address these issues, including vitamins and minerals, fish oil, digestive enzymes, and probiotics.

The first dietary step for Kate was removing all dairy. I have to admit that I was very skeptical that dietary changes would provide any major benefits to a child with autism, but we quickly saw huge improvements in her chronic gastrointestinal problems. Her bouts with diarrhea and constipation disappeared. A few months later we moved onto the second step by removing all gluten. We were told it could take several months for the gluten to be fully out of Kate's system, but we saw more immediate results and observed continued improvements extending well beyond the gastrointestinal issues. With gluten gone from Kate's system, we observed positive changes in her behavior and social interactions—we were amazed at the difference a gluten-free diet made.

She was also exhibiting fewer quirky and obsessive behaviors that I refer to as "autistic tendencies." These included toe walking and arm flapping, fixation or staring at objects, and "stimming." She even began to make progress in her ability to look at people when she was speaking with them and appeared to be much less withdrawn from her environment. It became obvious that the dietary changes and supplements we were experimenting with had made major improvements in all areas of her life. In time, even the chronic asthma her primary care physician diagnosed her with at age two had completely disappeared. We never thought that nutritional changes could make such a positive impact on Kate's quality of life. During this period, we were also continuing with all of Kate's additional therapies recommended by the NDP. Every small step in progress was a huge victory.

Additional tests from our environmental doctor later revealed increased levels of heavy metals and other chemicals present in Kate's blood and urine. We were instructed to minimize chemical stress on her body and made more dietary changes. We eliminated all food additives, preservatives, and artificial colorings and flavors—which we had already begun to do—and ensured that all her food was GMO-free. This meant no processed food, but only whole food sources. We bought mostly organically grown produce to minimize pesticide exposure. Embracing these changes was hard for a three-year-old, as it meant eating only the foods I cooked for her. Kate couldn't eat the usual foods offered at preschool school snack time, or at any birthday party, or at any family holiday gathering. Dining out at restaurants as a family and convenient drive-thru Happy Meals were never viable options. All of her meals had to be carefully prepared.

Our environmental doctor also explained how Kate was being exposed to toxic chemicals other than those found in food. We had to be vigilant in reading the labels on everything Kate came into contact with. Anything from personal care products, such as soap, shampoo, and toothpaste to over-the-counter (OTC) medications, could potentially contain harmful chemical ingredients confounding many of her autistic tendencies and disrupting the normal functioning of her body and mind. We removed any product used or consumed by Kate that contained toxic chemicals, and we modified her dental care (no fluoride and no silver fillings containing mercury). For this huge undertaking we found help on the websites and organizations already recommended in this book, including The Good Guide and The Environmental Working Group.

After much research, we decided that Kate would no longer receive any vaccines. This was a difficult choice, since my father and one brother are family doctors and another brother is a pediatrician. By this point, I'd learned so much about the intricate sensitivities of the immune system that I decided it wouldn't be in her best interest to receive vaccines and all of the chemical adjuvants they contained. Our primary care pediatrician did vaccine titers on Kate that tested the immunity levels in her body to the vaccines she'd already received. The immunity from her previous vaccines was still viable in her body more than two years **after** she was originally due for her boosters. If we hadn't done the titers and she'd received a booster on schedule, this could have potentially overloaded her sensitive immune system even further. It was obvious that for her, the vaccine risks outweighed the vaccine benefits. Children without Kate's sensitivities may warrant another decision.

From this point on, Kate's progress was dramatic. Her body and mind responded well to the elimination of many dangerous chemicals and other toxins in her diet, in our home, and in some traditional medical practices. We'd uncovered the root of many of her problems and were able to restore her health. By the time she was five, everyone we knew, including her primary care pediatrician, commented on the transformation they'd witnessed and by the time she reached seven, an independent NPD formally removed her label of autism. This was indeed something to celebrate!

The NDP's only concern for Kate was impulse control. For this we've found that chiropractic treatment, especially cranial manipulation (Koren-Specific-Technique), as well as drug-free homeopathic remedies (under the care of a homeopathic practitioner), have been extremely beneficial. After these treatments, Kate's impulsiveness improved considerably. At one point, when Kate was about five, we did follow the advice of the NDP and started ADHD medications. However, escalating behaviors and confounding side effects of the initial drugs resulted in the recommendation of a powerful antipsychotic. It was at this very low point that we stopped all medication and began looking for alternative, all natural therapies.

We're often asked what we credit for Kate's amazing recovery. This is a difficult and complicated question, because we used so many therapies to influence her well-being, both traditional and complementary. But I truly believe that the most significant benefits were gained from the practices found in environmental medicine, dietary changes, constitutional homeopathy, and chiropractic care (KST-specific therapy).

We're extremely grateful that our efforts and our diligence in fighting back against autism have improved the outlook for Kate's quality of life. It was far from easy, and for that reason, it's often the road less traveled. There is no quick fix for these children. For us, it demanded major changes in our lifestyle and forced us back to a more basic, natural, and holistic way of living and eating. There was also a huge financial burden associated with trying to improve a chronic illness with methods that rely heavily on all natural, organic, and specialty diet foods, nontoxic products, and integrative health practices not always covered by health insurance.

When Kate's life and health started going really well, my husband (and many other outsiders) often wondered is all this really necessary? Can't we pull back a little on how strict we are with her diet and toxin-free environment? My answer to this was an emphatic, "No!" Every time Kate now has some type of dietary or chemical infraction, it gives us a window into the chaotic world we'd still be living in if we weren't using the resources we're so blessed to have found. These infractions have resulted in temper tantrums, gastrointestinal problems, impulsiveness, and a poignant decline in mental wellness, moments that remind us that Kate's condition is chronic. If we don't monitor her diet and chemical insults, we feel certain that many of her prior challenges would return. This reinforces for us that all we're doing is still necessary for her to have the life she now has.

Kate's autism taught me to respect the human body and everything we put into it. It's also taught me how the human body has the capacity to help heal itself in very natural ways, through a simple recipe: nurture it with what it needs and take away things that harm it. For Kate, the daily solutions that ended up working were the most natural and common sense approaches found in environmental medicine and other complementary and integrative health practices. These alternative therapies carefully and thoughtfully treated all aspects of Kate, providing a gentle response to what her mind, body, and spirit were calling for.

Our success story would not have been possible without the support we received from other courageous autism parents who paved the way before us. They were our lifeline, encouraging us to ask questions, to continually search for answers, to follow our instincts, and to explore (under a doctor's supervision) whatever new methods were out there that might prove helpful. The support of others and our continual striving to learn all we could empowered us to help heal our daughter. Every unique journey helps to widen this road less traveled just a little more. I hope our story and the important information contained in this book can help awaken and inspire more mothers to set out on their own path to find answers so that every child's true voice can be heard.

Chapter 9

POLITICS

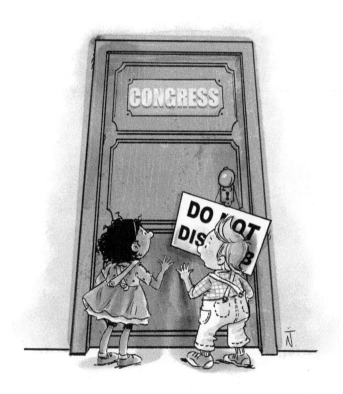

*The defeat of democracy and the end of the American
Revolution will occur when government falls into the hands
of the lending institutions and moneyed incorporations.*
—Thomas Jefferson (this notorious quote is paraphrased
from an 1825 letter to William Branch Giles)

MUSTERING POLITICAL WILLPOWER (JOANNE)

I never imagined I would have any interest in politics—until now. My personal experience with Patrick's cancer and my research for this book have opened my eyes to just how important our laws really are. The facts are undeniable. Until laws change, toxic chemicals known to cause cancer will remain pervasive in our environment, and far too many people will suffer needlessly. Our greatest hope for cancer lies not in a cure, but in having the political willpower to establish meaningful chemical reforms that can prevent this devastating disease from ever happening in the first place.

O ur children's health issues won't be fully addressed until we deal with the one final issue that underlies them all: our broken political system. Just the mere mention of the word "politics" can cause people to cringe and steer clear. Many of us have become far too removed from our political system, and as you have seen throughout this book, this disconnect is having a detrimental effect on the health of our children. If we want to see real change, change that puts children's health, well-being, and safety at the forefront of state and federal legislation, we need to "wake up" to what is happening in the political arena.

Complicating this task are common practices such as loopholes and piggyback legislation that often keep us from understanding the real impact a law may actually have in our society. Let's take a quick look at just a few of these practices playing out behind closed doors in our federal and state governments so we can be more informed.

Section 1: Political Practices Impeding Transparency

We may have democracy or we may have wealth concentrated
in the hands of a few, but we cannot have both.
—Justice Louis Brandeis

Lobbyists

In simple terms, lobbyists strive to influence the laws and policies of government at any level. They're usually hired by large corporations, trade associations, labor unions, or other special interest groups and paid to impact legislation affecting their particular business or interest. They frequently meet with lawmakers, regulatory agencies, judges, and even the President to influence the lawmaking process. Most of us know that corporations spend millions of dollars in lobbying efforts to protect their interest (which usually includes less regulation and less government oversight), but it's important to recognize that nonprofits and consumer groups also use lobbyists. For example, if legislation is about to be introduced for legalizing a new tobacco product, both sides of the issue will hire lobbyists to try to have the legislation either passed, blocked, or weakened. The practice raises concern of fairness when one side can afford to spend a lot more money on influencing policies and laws than another side. Should those with more money be afforded a louder and more influential voice in politics than those with less money?

Law Loopholes

A law loophole exempts specific people or groups or businesses from actually having to follow various aspects of the law. Loopholes are often written into a piece of legislation so that special interest groups are granted exceptions from that law. For example, we hear on the news that a wonderful policy was signed into law that considerably reduces the amount of toxic pollution released by industries into our environment. What we don't hear is that the same law contains a large loophole allowing "pollution permits" to be purchased by a select large and powerful industry. The loophole allows that industry to continue to exceed the pollution limits of the law by simply purchasing a permit to do so, while we're led to believe real change is taking place. Don't we deserve more transparency?

Piggyback Legislation

Piggyback legislation is also known as a "rider"—a law added on to the main piece of legislation, but often *completely unrelated*. This is a common tactic used to avoid the scrutiny of the main piece of legislation being voted on. For instance, a healthcare bill can include a government takeover of the student loan program so when one votes to pass the main healthcare legislation, which needs to be publicly debated, one automatically votes to pass the unrelated government student loan legislation. It's often used as a way to make something law quickly that wouldn't necessarily be passed on its own merit. Piggyback legislation is also commonly used in political party warfare to block or delay a law from being passed by attaching something unattractive to it. As a result, significant changes to our laws are being made without public input or legislative accountability. It's a perfectly legal, but sneaky tactic affecting the transparency of the legislative process and our right to know about and debate proposed laws. Other countries, such as France, Great Britain, and Hungary, do not permit piggyback legislation in their lawmaking branches.

Revolving Doors

A "revolving door" in political speak refers to how easy it is to move back and forth between a high-level job in industry and a high-level job in the government agency that oversees that same industry. There is also a "revolving door" between lawmakers and lobbyists who work for industry to influence lawmakers. For example, a former attorney who worked for an agricultural biotech company that created one of the first GMO food crops left the industry and went to work for the FDA. At the FDA, he helped to develop its GMO policy, declaring that GMO foods are "generally regarded as safe" (GRAS), and then he later wrote the policy that exempted GMO foods from labeling laws. After these policies were written, he left the FDA and eventually ended up working again for the same agricultural biotech company promoting genetically modified food. Revolving doors lead to potential conflicts of interest and corruption. Will the best interest of the public or the industry be served when former leaders of industry are now in positions as government regulators?

Food Libel Laws

Thirteen agriculture-friendly states have passed laws that make it either a criminal or civil offense to falsely accuse any food grower, producer, and/or manufacturer of harmful or tainted products. This may seem fair on the surface, but large and powerful food companies with lots of money now have the ability to sue anyone who says anything negative regarding their food product (even if it's true). If you talk about a specific food in a derogatory way, you risk being sued and may have to prove in court that *your accusations were accurate*, costing you thousands (if not millions) of dollars, even if you win your case——a far cry from the First Amendment freedoms established under our Constitution. One well-known example of food libel laws in action was the Texas Beef Group vs. Oprah Winfrey (N.D. Tex, CV-208-J). Oprah won the lawsuit filed against her for speaking out and exposing some of the problems within the beef industry. But it cost her in excess of a million dollars to defend her accurate statements about the industry in a court of law. Is this a fair and balanced practice? How will the public continue to be informed if laws like this exist?

Section 2: We the People or We the Corporations?

Let us not seek the Republican answer or the Democratic answer, but the right answer. Let us not seek to fix the blame for the past. Let us accept our responsibility for the future.
—John F. Kennedy

FINDING COMMON GROUND AS PARENTS (CHRISTINE)

Like Joanne, I never thought I would find myself involved in politics. However, over the last few years as environmental health threats became very real for my family and my community I had to find the courage to speak out.

As I walked to the front of the tension-filled room to speak at a public hearing for the proposed hazardous waste site in my area, I could feel my stomach tighten. The stakes could not be higher and tempers were flaring on both sides. I passed by a vocal group of union workers holding their signs high. They were fighting for jobs. I was there with a local grassroots environmental group fighting to protect our river, the source of drinking water for millions of people in our area now threatened by the proposed hazardous waste site. As I took the microphone my hands were shaking, and I began to share my personal story about Kaleigh and her chemical sensitivities. I also shared current statistics showing that our county was the only county in our state where pediatric cancer rates were rising. I looked out into the crowd as I closed and spoke from my heart "I think we all try to be good parents, all of us." Looking directly at the union members with respect I continued, "Yes, we do need jobs, but it cannot be at the expense of our children's health or our environment. What kind of society doesn't protect its children?" With that statement, I felt the room grow quiet. I realized that despite our differences, something as simple as love for our children can be the political common ground we need to build on.

An astronomical amount of money is now infiltrating our political system. Best-selling author, spiritual teacher, and political activist Marianne Williamson described our broken political system with the following words: "Moneyed forces now wield an influence on our political functioning totally disproportionate to the influence wielded by the average American citizen." For years big businesses have been fighting for (and winning) more rights and more power in our democracy, rights and power originally guaranteed to the "people" under the Constitution and Bill of Rights. Many Americans are completely unaware that in 2010 we suffered one of the greatest blows to our democracy in the Supreme Court ruling of Citizens United vs. the Federal Election Commission (FEC). This granted corporations the same First Amendment speech protection that people receive— and corporations were given the same rights to influence political elections as people. Are corporations really "people?"

Corporations are now able to donate billions of dollars to fund a politician or presidential candidate and remain *anonymous*. It's then a small step for elected officials to serve the needs of a corporation that helped elect them instead of the needs of the "people"—and certainly instead of the needs of our children. About 85 percent of Americans feel that corporations already have too much influence in our democracy. When did *we the people* become *we the corporations*? When did we forget that part of the duty of the people is to hold government *accountable*? As Americans awaken to the 2010 Supreme Court ruling in Citizens United, many have joined together to do something to change all this. Move to Amend is just one of the many grassroots organizations working towards a Constitutional amendment to get the money out of our political system and restore our democracy so that government can once again serve the people.

Practical Tools: What Can We Do?

You can join or support the many consumer advocacy groups and grassroots movements already involved in political action affecting the health of our children. Information on national efforts to strengthen protections for our children under various laws and many other political resources are conveniently located in the Resource Guide (see Part 3 or www.behindcloseddoorsthebook. com). Most organizations will keep you up-to-date on laws impacting our children and provide simple ways you can voice your support for or against laws by signing online petitions or letters to lawmakers. We also included organizations in the Resource Guide that are dedicated to reforming many of our current political processes, amending some of our laws, and getting money out of politics.

THROUGH THE EYES OF OUR CHILDREN (AMANDA)

When I first met Joanne and Christine, I was immediately inspired by their vision for a safer world for children. Although my two sons haven't experienced any chronic illnesses, I have one of those sensitive constitutions that feels the "sum of the parts" of all the low-level toxins in our world very clearly.

At the same time, I was also challenged: I agreed that moms should be relieved of the huge burden of having to navigate through so many potential dangers to their children, but I hated the idea of getting involved in politics. Everyone seems motivated by greed and selfishness, and the lowest-common-denominator candidate always seems to win. But then I began to think about it: maybe politics was this way precisely **because** mothers were not involved. Perhaps the best way to change our world was not to ignore politics, but to speak up. To go public with our love and common sense.

Since then, I've looked at every issue through the eyes of our children and the kind of world I want them to grow up in, and I've found a lot more motivation to speak up. I've become convinced there is no force more powerful than a mother's love, and to withhold it from public life is to withhold one of the purest and greatest forces for good the world has.

Section 3: United We Stand for Change

Never doubt that a small group of thoughtful committed citizens can change the world, Indeed, it is the only thing that ever has.
—Margaret Mead

It can be difficult to accept all that's been uncovered in this book. For too long many of us remained unaware of what's been playing out in many of our country's industries and affecting our children's health. Children don't have the power, money, or influence that big businesses have in our political system. Who will speak out on their behalf if we don't? Weak laws that govern our food (such as GRAS) and our chemicals (such as TSCA) desperately need more reform. For decades now, new chemicals and food additives have been introduced into products that reached our homes and our children without any real safety testing required, the very same chemicals and additives that are often banned in other countries. As our children's health statistics continue to worsen and autism rates continue to soar, we all need to sound the alarm and speak out politically on behalf of our children. Who will be our future teachers, nurses, firefighters, military, and workers in so many other professions if an increasing number of our children become disabled adults? It doesn't matter which political party you belong to because the common bond is our collective desire to love, nurture, and protect our children. It's up to all of us to stand together despite our differences, and become the voice of change for our children.

We *can* correct our current course by demanding laws that protect the health of our children and guarantee integrity, accountability, and transparency in industry practices. Never underestimate the power we hold as mothers, parents, and citizens banding together for one purpose. The pure intention of love we hold in our hearts for our children and their future can inspire action and fuel change quicker than we may realize. Author Margaret Wheatley best sums up how this happens and the power we ultimately hold in an excerpt from her book, *Turning to One Another: Simple Conversations to Restore Hope to the Future*:

> Large and successful change efforts start with conversations among friends, not with those in power: 'Some friends and I starting talking . . . ' Change doesn't happen from a leader announcing the plan. Change begins from deep inside a system, when a few people notice something they will no longer tolerate, or respond to a dream of what is possible. We just have to find a few others who care about the same thing. Together we will figure out what our first step is, then the next, then the next. Gradually, we become large and powerful. We don't have to start with power, only with passion.

Throughout our history we've seen many movements for social equality and racial justice, movements for various human rights causes that brought about important change and reformation. We saw the coming together of people for a common purpose and a common goal. These movements each began with a few visionaries, not the majority, inspiring others to imagine, to believe, to hope, that another possibility and a better way existed.

Imagine what our lives would be like if we all decided to envision a better system of protection for our children. We're standing at a new crossroads in our history where we must decide if we're going to sit by and silently watch our children's health continue to decline, or if we're going to join together to create the political changes that have become necessary. Changes that make children's health and wellness a top priority and that use children as the new measuring stick for clean air, clean water, and chemical safety. Let's embrace our power and let our children's voice be heard through us. They're calling us to action. How will we answer them?

Epilogue

COMING FULL CIRCLE

Just when the caterpillar thought the world was over, it became a butterfly.
—Unknown

As many of us know, when undertaking any type of project or endeavor there are unexpected obstacles and challenges we can't anticipate. Throughout the process of writing this book we were faced with our fair share of twists and turns. But little did we know we were both about to be blindsided once again by challenges to our children's health that also seriously jeopardized the completion of this book. We now realize that all we had learned along the way prepared us well for what we were about to undertake.

NEW CHALLENGE, NEW HEALING (CHRISTINE)

In the fall of 2012, I began to notice that Kaleigh was losing small patches of hair, and I immediately thought it was the result of her wearing her ponytail too tight. I called Joanne and asked if she knew about anything else that could cause this hair loss. After doing some research, she told me about an autoimmune condition called alopecia. When I said that I hope this wasn't what was happening to Kaleigh, she replied, "I hope not, either, because there doesn't appear to be any promising treatments."

I took Kaleigh to our family doctor and she did, in fact, diagnose her with alopecia, a rare autoimmune condition, but didn't know how to stop it from progressing or treat it. She said that all of Kaleigh's blood work was normal, which was a great relief, but she was at a loss for what was causing the alopecia. I thought of Patrick and all he had endured and this helped me keep perspective, yet I knew that this condition was extremely difficult for anyone to handle, especially an adolescent girl.

Within a few months, Kaleigh began losing large amounts of hair. She was having trouble maintaining normalcy at school, once her friends and peers began to notice this change as more and more of her hair fell out. I vividly remember Kaleigh sitting at our dining room table as I stood behind her trying to salvage what little hair she had left, which was knotted and tangled. She was crying and she was angry, taking her frustrations out on me as I tried to untangle her last strands of hair without them falling out in my hand. I was crying too, but didn't want Kaleigh to see or hear this. She needed me to be her strength, her calm, and her reassurance. I began to pray for guidance.

"Please help me," I said. "You know the helplessness I feel right now. Please give me strength to help Kaleigh!"

I was also very close to both of my grandmothers that had passed away. I was missing them in this moment and wished they were here to help. They were mothers too and would have understood the desperation I felt. For a brief moment it was as if they were standing right beside me. As difficult as this time was, I continued to affirm in my heart that Kaleigh would be healed, that her hair would grow back fully, and that there was a reason for this challenge in our lives.

By February 2013, Kaleigh was twelve and had lost all of her beautiful, long, curly hair. Her eyebrows and eyelashes were also gone. She had an advanced form of alopecia known as alopecia universalis involving a total loss of scalp and body hair. The diagnosis can have far-reaching social and emotional effects for a girl soon to be entering middle school. According to current medical literature, there is no cure for any form of alopecia. Although spontaneous hair regrowth happens frequently in those suffering from lesser forms of alopecia, there is a low chance of hair regrowth in alopecia universalis.

I felt so helpless and my heart was breaking for Kaleigh. Our entire family suffered right alongside her. My husband made an appointment with a specialist at one of the best medical facilities on the East Coast, but, as I suspected, they had nothing to offer except possible steroid treatments. I was very reluctant to have Kaleigh take steroids, given her sensitivities, so I sought out another doctor who also practices environmental medicine and homeopathy. She confirmed my concerns about steroids and suggested we retest Kaleigh for a variety of allergies and food sensitivities and then pursue a natural path for healing.

Since alopecia is an autoimmune condition, I knew we had to build up Kaleigh's immune system and allow her body to heal itself, as we'd done before. In recent years, we'd veered away from her strict diet, except for food connected to her life-threatening peanut and seafood allergies. As she'd gotten older and more independent, she wasn't always under my watchful eye when it came to eating. I knew she wasn't avoiding certain foods she was sensitive to that included gluten and dairy. She was also no longer eating only organic whole foods without GMOs and chemical pesticides. With four children, our family life was full of school sports and activities, and while I tried to cook nutritious meals often, I knew I had to get back on track with Kaleigh's diet.

The new tests confirmed that she still had life-threatening peanut and seafood allergies, with a list of other food sensitivities. When I got the report, I began having flashbacks to when she was a baby and remembered her autoimmune reaction to her nine-month vaccinations. Back then, I sometimes found clumps of hair in her crib and it wasn't until we tried to heal Kaleigh through diet and integrative therapies that her hair started to grow in thick, healthy, and strong. This was no coincidence, and there had to be a connection to what was going on now. I knew what I had to do to help Kaleigh, and I began implementing a strict organic whole foods diet, along with supplements, vitamins, and a variety of integrative therapies, including acupuncture. I'd already watched Kaleigh's body heal itself once, and knew we could help her body do it again.

This time around it was very hard to maintain a clean diet for Kaleigh because she was constantly on the run. One of the big challenges was her sports schedule. Many weekends we were away at soccer tournaments. It is easy to grab pizza, pretzels, and hot dogs at tournaments, but for Kaleigh these conveniences were not viable options. I had to prepare her meals ahead of time and pack foods to ensure she maintained a proper diet for healing.

As difficult and challenging as this time was for Kaleigh and my entire family, I feel so blessed and grateful for all the support we received from other families, friends, and the staff at her school. Kaleigh also had the support of so many wonderful friends. Her close group of girlfriends were her rock and her protector. The acts of kindness we received are too long to list, but one stands out. After Kaleigh's eyebrows had fallen out, one of her girlfriends and her mother came by the house and picked Kaleigh up to go shopping. I never considered myself to be good at hair or makeup so I was extremely thankful that this mom and daughter shared their talents with us. Kaleigh got everything she needed to do her eyebrows and they taught her how to do it herself. When I saw Kaleigh with her eyebrows back—beaming with self confidence in front of me—it filled me with such relief and joy that I started to cry. Never underestimate acts of kindness that we may deem small, because they can make all the difference in the world to the person on the other end.

Two years have passed and against the odds Kaleigh has regained almost all of her hair, as well as her eyebrows and eyelashes. I believe that her healing had everything to do with changes in her diet, supplements to boost her immune system, the use of various complementary and integrative health practices, and our faith. I am so proud of my daughter because of the strength and courage she's shown through this very difficult ordeal. Even though alopecia presented obvious emotional stress and self-esteem challenges, she maintained a very active social life and played competitive soccer wearing a wig. She also continued to attend school, even after being bullied on social media due to her appearance. Her determined spirit was something to behold. Despite the many tears, she never once allowed this condition to stop her from doing anything. She rose above it all and has emerged a stronger and more compassionate person. This experience has also enabled Kaleigh and I to provided support and information to other children and their families who suffer from this condition.

ANYTHING IS POSSIBLE (JOANNE)

In the fall of 2012, Patrick had a sudden onset of weakness in his left leg and left arm as well as difficulty walking and using his left hand. His primary doctor ordered an MRI of his head as a precaution, but the initial evaluation indicated that it was likely just the progression of his neuropathy—one of the many side effects of chemo from years ago. Off we went for the MRI with no real concerns. Within an hour of the radiologist having read the MRI, the phone rang. I was blindsided by the news that Patrick's MRI revealed a finding in the brain stem on the right pons. This could explain all of the difficulties he was having with the left side of his body.

I was in shock because I knew that a brain stem brain tumor was devastating, but the fact that this would be his second tumor made it that much worse. Patrick couldn't undergo any more radiation to the brain, the most effective treatment. As a child, he'd been exposed to very high doses, amounts which would be unthinkable to give today. His best hope for treatment would not be an option, and chemotherapy was not very effective in most brain tumors. Within a couple of weeks, a neurologist confirmed my suspicions that due to the location in the brain, performing a biopsy would be too dangerous and could leave him paralyzed or blind.

"Looking at Patrick's film," she told me, "it appears to be a cancer due to his initial radiation. That's what makes sense with his history. This is the area of the brain that previously received the highest dose of radiation and as you know radiation can also cause cancer."

This was very tough to hear, although I knew it was always a possibility. My son's lifesaving treatment as child, for which we were extremely thankful, could now be the root cause of a new cancer. The doctor explained that it was not uncommon for childhood brain tumor survivors to have strokes later in life, due to the effects of treatment. An MRA of Patrick's brain was scheduled for the next day to see if the film would possibly reveal the aftereffects of a stroke.

"A stroke," the doctor said, "is your best case scenario vs. the other possibility that we are dealing with a mass."

I pressed her for next steps if nothing showed up on the MRA and a stroke was ruled out. She candidly told me that it wasn't an ideal situation because we wouldn't know for sure what we were dealing with (a cancerous or noncancerous tumor), but that chemotherapy would be an option that oncology would discuss with us.

"No," I immediately told her. "I won't put Patrick through more treatments. I will not go that route with him."

He couldn't have more radiation, and chemo was much less effective. I believed that if we were dealing with a recurrence he would live longer and with a better quality of life without chemo treatments. As part of my job as a pharmaceutical medical writer, I'd worked on cancer clinical trials. I knew the upside of treatments, but I also knew the downside and Patrick had been through enough.

"Let's hope something shows up on the MRA tomorrow and it proves to be a stroke," the doctor said. "Another brain MRI is scheduled in six weeks. We can then see how it progresses and take it from there."

Following the MRA of the brain, the phone never rang. No news was bad news and Patrick hadn't suffered a stroke. Once again, life seemed to stand still and my medical writing came to a halt. We were in a holding pattern until Patrick's next MRI. All my energy was focused on helping my son and I now felt strong and confident in my ability to do this because I'd learned so much through my school, my work, and the research for this book. I'd also seen firsthand how Christine had used a variety of holistic medical practices to help heal Kaleigh from so many of her autoimmune issues. I had also witnessed remarkable results in my own niece Kate when using these same practices to overcome the diagnosis of autism. I truly believed these modalities could help in many different ways, but I was also grounded in the scientific reality that this was possibly a brain stem tumor recurrence in a body already compromised by cancer.

When I called Christine to share my concerns, she said, "There are so many things out there that can help Patrick without causing his body any more harm. Never underestimate the healing power we hold within ourselves. Mind, body, and spirit—all three make up Patrick. He is more than a body. Our mind and spirit are much more powerful than we realize."

While I knew all this, I needed to hear it again and her words were very comforting.

"More than anything," she went on, "you have to hold true to the belief that Patrick is going to be okay."

I had to get my mind out of the limited thinking of the five senses, yet I also needed my brain to rationalize what I was undertaking. I knew that we are made up of energy. All matter is made up of energy. There is energy in everything, including our thoughts, our words, and our prayers—and this energy holds the power to affect change. The field of quantum physics knows this well and I myself knew how powerful the mind was. Just look at something as simple as the "placebo effect" and what it can do to influence healing. I began to weave together all that I'd learned about traditional medicine, complementary and integrative therapies, energy work, health psychology, and my faith. My husband's family had even experienced its own documented medical miracle: an unexplained "spontaneous remission" from stage four brain cancer—attributed to the healing hands of a small Catholic nun. I truly believed that Patrick could be healed and I set out on a course of thoughtful action to bring this to fruition over the next six weeks. In my view, traditional treatments held no real hope for Patrick so I took a leap of faith and went into exploratory mode. I refused to put any more toxic treatments into his body and set about finding a kinder, gentler way to heal. This was my son and I wasn't going to lose him.

Marty had been traveling so much for work that we'd had barely a moment to sit down and have a serious conversation about all that had unfolded over the past ten days. I had to let him know the course I wanted to follow and see if he agreed. He'd always been such a wonderful and supportive husband and father that I knew in my heart he would trust me, but I was pitching a hard sell—especially for my husband, who like things in black and white. When we finally got a chance to talk about Patrick's reality, we cried together. I shared all my thoughts and research and beliefs about the situation, while he listened intently. Marty is very practical and was grateful that I was taking complete control of the medical piece and happy that I was hopeful. But I also knew that he thought I was a little crazy and might be in a temporary fantasy land, thinking that all these different approaches could help our son. I completely understood because ten years ago I'd also have thought myself crazy.

I reiterated the importance of positive thoughts and the power of believing that anything is possible. I reminded him of the story of his cousin Noreen, who was healed from cancer that had spread throughout her brain and how Marty's own father, a Philadelphia homicide detective and a man who also saw things as black or white, told us that he would not have believed it if he hadn't seen it with his own eyes. I asked Marty to take that lesson in faith from his father, who'd just passed away, and hold it for Patrick.

During the next six months I began implementing a wide variety of holistic healing modalities, including mild clay detox baths, herbal tea detox, a diet focused on plant-based foods, constitutional homeopathic medicine, vitamins, minerals, and lots of energy work including KST-specific chiropractic care. Additionally, I fully embraced the power of the mind and spirit through daily positive thoughts, positive visualization, affirmations, and prayers for Patrick.

I was committed to researching every therapeutic tool we used for Patrick and would only utilize those that would not cause him any harm. I also wanted to see if any traditional medical therapies held hope without toxic effects. My research led me to shark cartilage, which I found to be promising because it contains proteins with properties that can stop the process of blood vessel development. Tumors need a network of blood vessels to survive and grow, so cutting off the tumor's blood supply starves it of nutrients, theoretically causing it to shrink or disappear. According to the National Cancer Institute, AE-941 is a purified form of shark cartilage that continues to be researched for use in a variety of medical conditions, including the treatment of cancer. Although it has yet to be proven effective in humans, several clinical trials are currently ongoing. I knew this supplement held no claims to cure anything, but if it held any potential and was not harmful, I thought it was worth a try and after consulting with a doctor, I added it to my son's regimen.

I told very few people about Patrick because I was concerned about what I would say and how they would respond. It wasn't a good scenario for conversation and I knew the importance of keeping out all negative thinking. I'd begun building a wall to shut out any distractions.

During Hurricane Sandy in the fall of 2012, Patrick's body began to show that he was responding to the mild detox. He had a cough, a runny nose, achiness, and fatigue. He also had discharge coming from both his ears. His homeopathic doctor had suggested mild detox after learning that we'd never been instructed to do any type of detoxification following Patrick's initial radiation and chemo. To her this defied taking care of the human body. Hurricane Sandy left us without power for a few days, which I found to be a blessing in disguise. No work. No TV. No computers. No running. I enjoyed the opportunity to stay at home and for Patrick's body to rest completely. Within a few days, all of his symptoms passed.

The next six weeks were challenging as I tried to hold strong to the vision of Patrick's tumor shrinking and of seeing him completely healed. I was not having a chemo conversation with an oncologist, but instead envisioning receiving good news. We kept to a strict routine of therapies.

A week before Patrick's next brain MRI, he appeared to be showing some signs of improvement. His left side was gaining a little strength and he felt steadier walking. I was ecstatic for any small signs of hope, letting me know all our efforts were not in vain. The day finally arrived and we went for our scheduled appointment with the neurologist at the Hospital of the University of Pennsylvania to find out the results of the MRI. I was beside myself with expectation and anxiety. But I also knew that I'd done all I could. I was at peace with that part and decided to put the results in God's hands.

Before going to the hospital, my son Colin came into my room and hugged me.

"Everything's going to be fine, Mom," he said. "I just know it."

My eyes filled up with tears and for the first time I allowed in some doubt and was braced for anything.

The neurology floor of the hospital was somewhat depressing, in part because there were so many patients in the waiting area with serious neurological disorders. I knew too well that their daily lives were a struggle not only for them, but for their families who cared for them. As we waited for our appointment, there was a toddler sitting on the floor in front of us joyfully playing with her toys. She was young, healthy, and vibrant and she gave me a burst of hope amidst the sense of silent desperation that filled the room. The wait was excruciating. I felt numb and as if I'd been holding my breath ever since I got the initial call about Patrick months earlier. I tried my best to make small talk with Marty and Patrick, until they finally called his name. My stomach sunk as we stood to walk down the long hallway. The doctor was waiting for us and the moment we stepped into the room she smiled.

"It's good news!" she proclaimed. "When I saw the MRI results, I couldn't believe it. Whatever was there has substantially decreased in size. We really don't know what to think because not only did it shrink, but there were also some areas of damage in the brain that showed up on his previous MRIs that are now also resolved."

I was overwhelmed by what I was hearing. I was elated and shot Marty an "I told you so" look across the room. I desperately wanted the doctor to ask us what we'd been doing for Patrick, but she didn't. Instead she said, "In essence, we don't really know what it is now, because as you know, cancer and tumors don't just go away."

I wanted to scream, "I believe anything is possible!" but I held back because Patrick wasn't totally healed.

Something very small remained on the right pons, so another MRI was scheduled in six months.

On the way to the elevator I was thrilled and excited, but still anxious over the news that could have resulted from that appointment. Marty and I were still numb as we went across the street to eat and celebrate with Patrick.

When we finally sat down, I said, "Can we recap what we just heard in there? I want to make sure I got it right."

"You did," Marty said. "Not only was the tumor almost gone, but previous trouble areas had also cleared up."

How do you explain that? I asked myself. I didn't know the answer for sure, but right now I felt as if I could finally exhale. I had so many people to call and thank, including all of the wonderful practitioners we were using. I first let my family know, then I phoned Christine who'd been suffering my agony right alongside me and was a great source of encouragement and strength. When I told her the good news, all she could do was cry. For the next six months, we continued our vigilance with all the therapies we were doing for Patrick and when we went back for his follow-up MRI in the spring, the initial finding on the right pons was completely gone. The doctor made it a point to stress how incredibly wonderful this news really was.

"Last fall when you walked through those doors," she said, "I thought we were headed down a very different path."

Then we received more good news. During his initial cancer treatments, Patrick suffered damage to the pituitary gland, leaving him adrenal insufficient and on steroids for many years. His adrenal glands are now working again and he's no longer on daily steroids for adrenal insufficiency. His last Dexa Scan performed for his steady progression of bone loss was also markedly improved without the use of any supplements.

Something was working that isn't found in medical textbooks. It is only found by going deep within yourself and discovering the courage to believe in a vision grander than the one before you and the strength to never stop looking for ways to get there.

Throughout this book, we have shared with you all we have learned through our own personal experiences with our children's health challenges. The journey was arduous at times, and it took perseverance and faith to continue on the path to find our own answers to the problems Patrick and Kaleigh faced. It has made us stronger in so many ways and empowered us to become *active participants* in our children's health and also in the communities we live in.

We hope that that it can awaken each of you to the power *you* hold in the choices you make. Never stop searching for answers when it comes to better health for your children. Always listen to your instincts and empower yourself by doing your own research. It will open doors to new possibilities that can make a difference for your child and may even help pave the way for others. As mothers and parents, we are indeed our children's greatest advocates and their strongest voice for change.

REFERENCES AND RESOURCE GUIDE

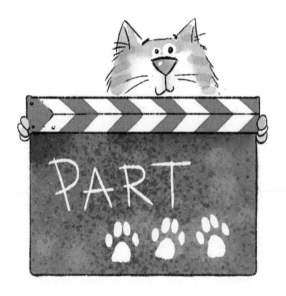

REFERENCES

Chapters 1 and 2

Food & Water Watch. *A Toxic Flood*. Food & Water Watch. May 16, 2013. Accessed August 2, 2013. http://www.foodandwaterwatch.org/reports/a-toxic-flood/.

Bean, Nancy H., PhD, Joy S. Goulding, Christopher Lao, and Frederick J. Angulo, DVM, PhD. "Surveillance for Foodborne-Disease Outbreaks—United States, 1988–1992." *CDC Morbidity and Mortality Weekly Report (MMWR)* 45, no. SS-5 (October 25, 1996): 1–55. http://www.cdc.gov/mmwr/preview/mmwrhtml/00044241.htm.

Belliveau, Michael E. "The Drive for a Safer Chemicals Policy in the United States." *New Solutions* 21, no. 3 (2011): 359–86. doi:10.2190/NS.21.3.e.

Biro, F. M., M. P. Galvez, L. C. Greenspan, P. A. Succop, N. Vangeepuram, S. M. Pinney, S. Teitelbaum, G. C. Windham, L. H. Kushi, and M. S. Wolff. "Pubertal Assessment Method and Baseline Characteristics in a Mixed Longitudinal Study of Girls." *Pediatrics* 126, no. 3 (2010): E583–590. Accessed August 28, 2012. doi:10.1542/peds.2009-3079.

"Bisphenol A (BPA)." National Institute of Environmental Health Sciences. Accessed June 12, 2013. http://www.niehs.nih.gov/news/sya/sya-bpa/index.cfm.

Blumberg, Stephen J., PhD, Matthew D. Bramlett, PhD, Michael D. Kogan, PhD, Laura Schieve, PhD, Jessica R. Jones, MPH, and Michael C. Lu, MD, MPH. "Changes in Prevalence of Parent-reported Autism Spectrum Disorder in School-aged U.S. Children: 2007 to 2011–2012." *National Health Statistics Report* 65 (March 20, 2013).

"Body Burden: The Pollution in Newborns." Environmental Working Group. July 2005. Accessed October 20, 2013. http://www.ewg.org/research/body-burden-pollution-newborns.

"Bovine Growth Hormone." Food Water Watch. Accessed August 23, 2012. https://www.foodandwaterwatch.org/food/foodsafety/dairy.

"CFC SB 772 Fact Sheet: Toxic Flame Retardants and Fire Safety Alternatives." Consumer Federation of California. August 12, 2007. http://consumercal.org/cfc-sb-772-fact-sheet-toxic-flame-retardants-and-fire-safety-alternatives/.

"Chemical Profile for BHT (2,6-DI-TERT-BUTYL-P-CRESOL) CAS Number: 128-37-0." Scorecard. Accessed June 01, 2015. http://scorecard.goodguide.com/about/about.tcl.

"Cleaning Up a Broken CFL." United States Environmental Protection Agency. N.p., n.d. Web. 01 June 2015.

"Common Ingredients in U.S. Licensed Vaccines." U.S. Food and Drug Administration. Accessed May 30, 2014. http://www.fda.gov/BiologicsBloodVaccines/SafetyAvailability/VaccineSafety/ucm187810.htm.

"Congress Must Act to Remove Toxic Substances from Products Our Families Use Everyday: Flame Retardants TDCP and TCEP." National Resources Defense Council. July 2010. Accessed August 30, 2013. http://www.nrdc.org/health/flameretardants-fs.asp.

Dabelea, Dana, MD, PhD. "SEARCH for Diabetes in Youth—an Extended Registry Study, with Numerous Substudies Examining a Wide Variety of Factors Associated with Types 1 and 2 Disease." Proceedings of American Diabetes Association's 72nd Scientific Session, Pennsylvania Convention Center, Philadelphia.

"Depression in Children Part 1." *Harvard Mental Health Newsletter* (February 2002): n. pag. Web. 18 Sept. 2012. http://www.health.harvard.edu/newsweek/Depression_in_Children_Part_I.html.

"Fact #1: No Health Tests Are Required by Law to Put a Chemical on the Market." Chemical Industry Archives, a Project of the Environmental Working Group. Accessed April 16, 2015. http://www.chemicalindustryarchives.org/factfiction/facts/1.asp.

Fiedler, Heidelore. *Dioxin and Furan Inventories National and Regional Emissions of PCDD/PCDF.* May 1999. United Nations Environment Programme (UNEP) Chemicals, Geneva, Switzerland. Available online at http://www.unep.org/chemicalsandwaste/portals/9/POPs/Toolkit-Inventories/difurpt.pdf.

"Formaldehyde." The American Cancer Society. Accessed September 23, 2015. http://www.cancer.org/cancer/cancercauses/othercarcinogens/intheworkplace/formaldehyde.

Gascon, Mireia, Marta Fort, David Martinez, Anne-Elie Carsin, Joan Forns, Joan O. Grimalt, Loreto Santa Marina, Nerea Lertxundi, Jordi Sunyer, and Martine Vrijheid. "Polybrominated Diphenyl Ethers (PBDEs) in Breast Milk and Neuropsychological Development in Infants." *Environmental Health Perspectives* 120, no. 12 (2012): 1760–765. doi:10.1289/ehp.1205266.

Hamilton, Jon. "Feds Reject Petition to Ban BPA in Food." NPR. March 30, 2012. http://www.npr.org/blogs/thesalt/2012/03/30/149683556/feds-to-decide-on-banning-bpa-from-food-and-other-products.

Jacobson, Michael F., PhD, and David Schardt, MS. *Diet, ADHD and Behavior: A Quarter Century of Review.* Report. Washington, DC: Center for Science in the Public Interest, 1999.

LeFever, Gretchen B., PhD, Andrea P. Arcona, and David O. Antonuccio. "ADHD among American Schoolchildren Evidence of Overdiagnosis and Overuse of Medication." *The Scientific Review of Mental Health Practice* 2, no. 1 (Spring/Summer 2003). http://www.srmhp.org/0201/adhd.html.

Lipman, Terri H., PhD, CRNP, Lorraine E. Levitt Katz, MD, Sarah J. Ratcliffe, PhD., Kathryn M. Murphy, PhD, RN, Alexandra Aguilar, MD, Iraj Rezvani, MD, Carol J. Howe, MSN, RN, Shruti Fadia, MD, and Elizabeth Suarez, MD. "Increasing Incidence of Type 1 Diabetes in Youth Twenty Years of the Philadelphia Pediatric Diabetes Registry." *Diabetes Care*, January 22, 2013. doi:10.2337/dc12-0767.

Meeting of the California Environmental Contaminant Biomonitoring Program Scientific Guidance Panel. 4–5 Dec. 2008. SGP Meeting. Meeting document accessed online at http://oehha. ca.gov/multimedia/biomon/pdf/120408flamedoc.pdf.

"Pollution Locator: USA." Scorecard. Accessed May 23, 2015. http://scorecard.goodguide.com/ env-releases/us-map.tcl.

Safer Chemicals, Healthy Families (Website 2013). Research. *Congress Must Act to Remove Toxic Substances From Products Our Families Use Everyday: Flame Retardants TDCP and TCEP.* Accessed August 30, 2013. http://www.saferchemicals.org/resources/chemicals/tdcp-tcep. html.

Scallan, Elaine, Patricia M. Griffin, Frederick J. Angulo, Robert V. Tauxe, and Robert M. Hoekstra. "Foodborne Illness Acquired in the United States—Unspecified Agents." *Emerging Infectious Diseases* 17, no. 1 (January 2011). doi:10.3201/eid1701.P21101.

Shogren, Elizabeth. "CFL Bulbs Have One Hitch: Toxic Mercury." NPR. March 15, 2007. http://www.npr.org/templates/story/story.php?storyId=7431198.

Sicherer, Scott H., Anne Muñoz-Furlong, James H. Godbold, and Hugh A. Sampson. "U.S. Prevalence of Self-reported Peanut, Tree Nut, and Sesame Allergy: 11-year Follow-up." *Journal of Allergy and Clinical Immunology* 125, no. 6 (2010): 1322–1326. doi:10.1016/j. jaci.2010.03.029.

Stefanidou, M., C. Maravelias, and C. Spiliopoulou. "Human Exposure to Endocrine Disruptors and Breast Milk." *Endocrine, Metabolic & Immune Disorders - Drug Targets* 9, no. 3 (September 2009): 269–76. doi:10.2174/187153009789044374.

The Story of Stuff. By Annie Leonard and Jonah Sachs. Directed by Louis Fox. Performed by Annie Leonard. Free Range Studios. December 2007. http://storyofstuff.org/movies/story-of-stuff/.

"Thimerosal in Vaccines." U.S. Food and Drug Administration. June 14, 2014. http://www.fda. gov/BiologicsBloodVaccines/SafetyAvailability/VaccineSafety/UCM096228#t1.

Tomljenovic, L., and C. Shaw. "Mechanisms of Aluminum Adjuvant Toxicity and Autoimmunity in Pediatric Populations." *Lupus* 21, no. 2 (2012): 223–30. doi:10.1177/0961203311430221.

"Toxicological Profile for Aluminum." Agency for Toxic Substances and Disease Registry (ATSDR). September 2008. http://www.atsdr.cdc.gov/toxprofiles/tp.asp?id=191&tid=34.

"Toxicological Profile for Formaldehyde." Agency for Toxic Substances and Disease Registry (ATSDR). July 1999. http://www.atsdr.cdc.gov/toxprofiles/tp.asp?id=220&tid=39.

"Toxicological Profile for Mercury." Agency for Toxic Substances and Disease Registry (ATSDR). March 1999. http://www.atsdr.cdc.gov/toxprofiles/tp.asp?id=115&tid=24.

U.S. Congress. House. Government Reform. *Mercury in Medicine—Taking Unnecessary Risks.* By Dan Burton. 106 Cong. H. Rept. 76. Vol. 149. Government Printing Office, 2003.

U.S. Congress. Senate. Subcommittee on Children and Families of the Committee on Health, Education, Labor, and Pensions. *Examining Childhood Obesity, Focusing on the Declining Health of America's Next Generation National Problem, Southern Crisis.* 110th Cong., 2d sess. S. Doc. S. HRG. 110-447. Washington: U.S. Printing Office, 2008.

U.S. Congress. Senate. Subcommittee on Superfund, Toxins, and Environmental Health of the Committee on Environment and Public Works. *Assessing the Effectiveness of U.S. Chemical Safety Laws.* 112th Cong., 1st sess. S. Doc. S. HRG. 112-819. Washington: U.S. Printing Office, 2011.

United Nations. Food and Agriculture Organization. *The Codex General Standard for the Labeling of Prepackaged Foods (CODEX STAN 1985).* Amended in 2010. Accessed March 21, 2013. http:/www.codexalimentarius.net.

United States. Centers for Disease Control and Prevention. National Center for Health Statistics. *Prevalence of Obesity Among Children and Adolescents: United States, Trends 1963–1965 Through 2007–2008*. By Cynthia Ogden, PhD, and Margaret Carroll, MSPH. Accessed April 28, 2010. http://www.cdc.gov/nchs/data/hestat/obesity_child_07_08/obesity_child_07_08.htm.

United States. Centers for Disease Control and Prevention. National Center for Health Statistics. *NCHS Data Brief: Trends in Asthma Prevalence, Health Care Use, and Mortality in the United States, 2001–2010*. By Lara J. Akinbami, MD, Jeanne E. Moorman, MS, Cathy Bailey, MS, Hatice S. Zahran, MD, Michael King, PhD, Carol A. Johnson, MPH, and Xiang Liu, MS. May 2012. www.cdc.gov/nchs/data/databriefs/db94.pdf.

United States. Centers for Disease Control and Prevention. National Center for Health Satistics. *NCHS Data Brief: Recent Trends in Infant Mortality in the United States*. By Marion F. MacDorman, PhD, and T. J. Mathews, MS. October 2008. Accessed April 15, 2010. http://www.cdc.gov/nchs/data/databriefs/db09.pdf.

United States. Centers for Disease Control and Prevention. Office of Analysis and Epidemiology. *The State of Childhood Asthma, United States, 1980–2005*. By Lara J. Akinbami, MD. Vol. 381. Hyattsville, MD: NCHS, 2006.

United States. Central Intelligence Agency. *Online World Factbook: Infant Mortality Rate Country Comparison* Accessed January 22, 2015. https://www.cia.gov/library/publications/the-world-factbook/rankorder/2091rank.html.

United States. Department of Health and Human Services. National Cancer Institute. *Reducing Environmental Cancer Risk, What We Can Do Now—2008–2009 Annual Report President's Cancer Panel*. By Suzanne H. Reuben. April 2010. http://deainfo.nci.nih.gov/advisory/pcp/annualReports/pcp08-09rpt/PCP_Report_08-09_508.pdf.

United States. Department of Education. National Center for Education Statistics. *The Condition of Education 2010, NCES 2010 - 028*. By Aud, Susan, William Hussar, Michael Planty, Thomas Snyder, Kevin Bianco, Mary Ann Fox, Lauren Frohlich, Jana Kemp, and Lauren Drake. May 2010. http://nces.ed.gov/pubs2010/2010028.pdf.

United States. Department of Education. National Center for Education Statistics. *The Condition of Education 2012*, NCES 2012-045. By Susan Aud, William Hussar, Frank Johnson, Grace Kena, Erin Roth, Eileen Manning, Xiaolei Wang, and Jijun Zhang. May 2012. http://nces.ed.gov/pubs2012/2012045.pdf.

United States. Department of Agriculture. Economic Research Service. USDA *ERS—Adoption of Genetically Engineered Crops in the U.S.: Recent Trends in GE Adoption*. Accessed May 03, 2015. http://www.ers.usda.gov/data-products/adoption-of-genetically-engineered-crops-in-the-us/recent-trends-in-ge-adoption.aspx#.VDrS2Pn.

"Update on Bisphenol A (BPA): Use in Food Contact Application." U.S. Food and Drug Administration. November 2014. http://www.fda.gov/NewsEvents/PublicHealthFocus/ucm064437.htm#regulations.

Van Cleave, J., S. L. Gortmaker, and J. M. Perrin. "Dynamics of Obesity and Chronic Health Conditions Among Children and Youth." *JAMA: The Journal of the American Medical Association* 303, no. 7 (2010): 623–30. doi:10.1001/jama.2010.104.

"Video: 10 Americans." Environmental Working Group. July 23, 2012. Accessed October 20, 2013. http://www.ewg.org/news/videos/10-americans.

Weil, Elizabeth. "Puberty Before Age 10: A New 'Normal'?" *The New York Times*, March 30, 2012. http://www.nytimes.com/2012/04/01/magazine/puberty-before-age-10-a-new-normal.html?pagewanted=2&_r=3.

World Health Organization. International Agency for Research on Cancer. *IARC Monographs on the Evaluation of Carcinogenic Risks to Humans.* Vol. 40. BHT Pages 161–206. Lyon, France: International Agency for Research on Cancer, 1986.

Writing Group for the SEARCH for Diabetes in Youth Study Group, D. Dabelea, R. A. Bell, R. B. D'Agostino, Jr, G. Imperatore, J. M. Johansen, B. Linder, L. L. Liu, B. Loots, S. Marcovina, E. J. Mayer-Davis, D. J. Pettitt, and B. Waitzfelder. "Incidence of Diabetes in Youth in the United States." *JAMA: The Journal of the American Medical Association* 297, no. 24 (June 27, 2007): 2716-724. doi:10.1001/jama.297.24.2716.

Yum, Taewoo, Sanghouck Lee, and Yunje Kim. "Association between Precocious Puberty and Some Endocrine Disruptors in Human Plasma." *Journal of Environmental Science and Health, Part A: Toxic/Hazardous Substances and Environmental Engineering* 48, no. 8 (2013): 912–17. doi:10.1080/10934529.2013.762734.

Zarcone, Dana. "The Alarming Statistics on Childhood Depression." Ezine Articles. Accessed September 18, 2012. http://ezinearticles.com/?The-Alarming-Statistics-on-Childhood-Depression&id=4877622.

Chapter 3

"About Food Allergy." The Food Allergy and Anaphylaxis Network - FAAN. Accessed September 17, 2012. http://www.foodallergy.org/section/about-food-allergy.

Adamson, Peter. "Measuring Child Poverty: New League Tables of Child Poverty in the World's Rich Countries." UNICEF Innocenti Research Centre Report Card 10. Accessed September 12, 2012. http://www.unicef-irc.org/publications/660.

Allen, D. B. "Influence of Inhaled Corticosteroids on Growth: A Pediatric Endocrinologist's Perspective." *Acta Paediatrica* 87, no. 2 (February 1998): 123–29. doi:10.1111/j.1651-2227.1998.tb00960.x.

"Allergy Statistics." The American Academy of Allergy Asthma and Immunology. Accessed September 17, 2012. http://www.aaaai.org/about-the-aaaai/newsroom/allergy-statistics.aspx.

"Allergy Statistics." The American Academy of Allergy, Asthma, and Immunology. Accessed September 17, 2012. http://www.aaaai.org/about-the-aaaai/newsroom/allergy-statistics.aspx.

American Diabetes Association. "Diabetes Rates Increase Significantly Among American Youth." News release, June 9, 2012. Press Room. http://www.diabetes.org/for-media/2012/sci-sessions-SEARCH.html.

"Autism Prevalence Now 1 in 88 Children, 1 in 54 Boys." National Autism Association. Accessed June 5, 2013. http://nationalautismassociation.org/autism-prevalence-now-1-in-88-children-1-in-54-boys/.

"Autism Spectrum Disorders (ASDs)—Data & Statistics." Centers for Disease Control and Prevention. March 29, 2012. http://www.cdc.gov/ncbddd/autism/data.html.

"Autism: MedlinePlus Medical Encyclopedia." U.S National Library of Medicine. Accessed December 15, 2010. http://www.nlm.nih.gov/medlineplus/ency/article/001526.htm.

Bell, R. A., E. J. Mayer-Davis, J. W. Beyer, R. B. D'Agostino, J. M. Lawrence, B. Linder, L. L. Liu, S. M. Marcovina, B. L. Rodriguez, D. Williams, and D. Dabelea. "Diabetes in Non-Hispanic White Youth: Prevalence, Incidence, and Clinical Characteristics: The SEARCH for Diabetes in Youth Study." *Diabetes Care* 32, no. Supplement_2 (2009): S102-111. doi:10.2337/dc09-S202.

Bethell, C. D., M. D. Kogan, B. B. Strickland, E. L. Schor, J. Robertson, and P. W. Newacheck. "Academic Pediatrics. A National and State Profile of Leading Health Problems and Health Care Quality for US Children: Key Insurance Disparities and Across-state Variations." *Academic Pediatrics* 11, no. 3 (2011): Suppl. S22-33.

Biro, F. M., M. P. Galvez, L. C. Greenspan, P. A. Succop, N. Vangeepuram, S. M. Pinney, S. Teitelbaum, G. C. Windham, L. H. Kushi, and M. S. Wolff. "Pubertal Assessment Method and Baseline Characteristics in a Mixed Longitudinal Study of Girls." *Pediatrics* 126, no. 3 (2010): E583–590. Accessed August 28, 2012. doi:10.1542/peds.2009-3079.

Blumberg, Stephen J., PhD, Matthew D. Bramlett, PhD, Michael D. Kogan, PhD, Laura Schieve, PhD, Jessica R. Jones, MPH, and Michael C. Lu, MD, MPH. "Changes in Prevalence of Parent-reported Autism Spectrum Disorder in School-aged U.S. Children: 2007 to 2011–2012." *National Health Statistics Report* 65 (March 20, 2013). http://www.cdc.gov/nchs/data/nhsr/nhsr065.pdf.

Bock, Kenneth, Cameron Stauth, and Korri Fink. *Healing the New Childhood Epidemics: Autism, ADHD, Asthma, and Allergies: The Groundbreaking Program for the 4-A Disorders*. New York: Ballantine Books, 2007. 124–26; 142–145.

Bouchard, M. F., D. C. Bellinger, R. O. Wright, and M. G. Weisskopf. "Attention-Deficit/ Hyperactivity Disorder and Urinary Metabolites of Organophosphate Pesticides." *Pediatrics* 125, no. 6 (2010): E1270–1277. doi:10.1542/peds.2009-3058.

Boyle, C. A., S. Boulet, L. A. Schieve, R. A. Cohen, S. J. Blumberg, M. Yeargin-Allsopp, S. Visser, and M. D. Kogan. "Trends in the Prevalence of Developmental Disabilities in US Children, 1997-2008." *Pediatrics* 127, no. 6 (2011): 1034–042. doi:10.1542/peds.2010-2989.

Branum, A. M., and S. L. Lukacs. "Food Allergy Among Children in the United States." *Pediatrics* 124, no. 6 (December 2009): 1549–555. doi:10.1542/peds.2009-1210.

Cancer Facts and Figures 2014, Special Section: Cancer in Children and Adolescents. 2014. American Cancer Society, Atlanta.

"CDC Estimates 1 in 88 Children in United States Has Been Identified as Having an Autism Spectrum Disorder." News release. Centers for Disease Control and Prevention. Accessed September 26, 2012. http://www.cdc.gov/media/releases/2012/p0329_autism_disorder.html.

Centers for Disease Control and Prevention. Accessed September 17, 2012. http://www.cdc.gov/nchs/fastats/adhd.htm.

Centers for Disease Control and Prevention. Accessed September 29, 2010. http://www.cdc.gov/healthyyouth/obesity/.

Centers for Disease Control and Prevention. Accessed March 21, 2016. http://www.cdc.gov/reproductivehealth/maternalinfanthealth/infantmortality.htm.

Centers for Disease Control and Prevention. National Center for Chronic Disease Prevention & Health Promotion. "CDC Funds Registries for Childhood Diabetes." News release, November 21, 2000. CDC. http://www.cdc.gov/media/pressrel/r2k1226.htm.

"Childhood Cancer Statistics." American Childhood Cancer Organization. Accessed August 27, 2012. http://www.acco.org/Information/AboutChildhoodCancer/ChildhoodCancerStatistics.aspx.

"Children and Diabetes — More Information." Centers for Disease Control and Prevention. April 03, 2012. Accessed September 15, 2012. http://www.cdc.gov/diabetes/projects/cda2.htm.

"Chronic Arthropathy Associated with Rubella Vaccination." *Arthritis & Rheumatism* 20, no. 2 (November 2005): 741–47.

Classen, J. B. "Association between Type 1 Diabetes and Hib Vaccine." *British Medical Journal* 319 (1999): 1133.

Committing to Child Survival: A Promise Renewed. September 2012. Progress Report 2012, Division of Policy and Strategy, UNICEF, 3 United Nations Plaza, New York, NY.

Dabelea, Dana, MD, PhD. "SEARCH for Diabetes in Youth–an Extended Registry Study, with Numerous Substudies Examining a Wide Variety of Factors Associated with Types 1 and 2 Disease." Proceedings of American Diabetes Association's 72nd Scientific Session, Pennsylvania Convention Center, Philadelphia.

"Depression in Children Part 1." *Harvard Mental Health Newsletter*, February 2002. Accessed September 18, 2012. http://www.health.harvard.edu/newsweek/Depression_in_Children_Part_I.htm.

Deshmukh, CT. "Minimizing Side Effects of Systemic Corticosteroids in Children." *Indian Journal of Dermatology, Venereology and Leprology* 73, no. 4 (2007): 218–21. doi:10.4103/0378-6323.33633.

Evertsen, Jennifer, Ramin Alemzadeh, and Xujing Wang. "Increasing Incidence of Pediatric Type 1 Diabetes Mellitus in Southeastern Wisconsin: Relationship with Body Weight at Diagnosis." Edited by Adrian Vella. *PLoS ONE* 4, no. 9 (2009): E6873. doi:10.1371/journal.pone.0006873.

"Food Allergy Resources." Kids with Food Allergies—KFA. Accessed May 12, 2012. http://www.kidswithfoodallergies.org/resourcespre.php?id=62.

"Food Allergy Resources." Kids with Food Allergies–KFA. Accessed May 12, 2012. http://www.kidswithfoodallergies.org/resourcespre.php?id=62.

"General LD Info." The National Center for Learning Disabilities. Accessed September 26, 2012. http://www.ncld.org/types-learning-disabilities/what-is-ld.

Georgiou, George J., PhD, DSc (AM), ND. "A Natural Heavy Metal Chelator Is Born." *British Naturopathic Journal* 24, no. 1 (2007): 14–17. http://www.detox-heavymetals.com/docs/British_Naturopathic_Journa.pdf.

Gewanter, Harry L., Klaus J. Roghmann, and John Baum. "The Prevalence of Juvenile Arthritis." *Arthritis & Rheumatism* 26, no. 5 (1983): 599–603. doi:10.1002/art.1780260504.

Glenn D., MD. "Is 7 the New 10? Why Do Some Girls Start Puberty So Early?" *Huffington Post (blog)*, August 27, 2012. http://www.huffingtonpost.com/glenn-d-braunstein-md/early-puberty_b_1826072.html.

Guardasil (Human Papillomavirus Quadrivalent (Types 6, 11, 16, and 18) Vaccine, Recombinant. Full Prescribing Information, Merck and Co., Inc. Accessed online at: http://www.merck.com/product/usa/pi_circulars/g/gardasil/gardasil_pi.pdf.

HCCI. "Press Release: Children's Health Care Spending Report 2007-2010." News release, July 1, 2012. Health Care Cost Institute. Accessed September 18, 2012. http://www.healthcostinstitute.org/news-and-events/press-release-childrens-health-care-spending-report-2007-2010.

Herman-Giddens, Marcia E., PA, MPH, DrPH, Jennifer Steffes, MSW, Donna Harris, MA, Eric Slora, PhD, Michael Hussey, MS, Steven A. Dowshen, MD, Richard Wasserman, MD, MPH, Janet R. Serwint, MD, Lynn Smitherman, MD, and Edward O. Reiter, MD. "Secondary Sexual Characteristics in Boys: Data from the Pediatric Research in Office Settings Network." *Pediatrics*, October 20, 2012. doi: 10.1542/peds.2011-3291.

Howson, Christopher P., Cynthia J. Howe, and Harvey V. Fineberg. *Adverse Effects of Pertussis and Rubella Vaccines.* Washington, DC: National Academy Press, 1991. 187–88.

Jacobson, Michael F., PhD, and David Schardt, M.S. *Diet, ADHD and Behavior: A Quarter Century of Review.* Report. Washington, DC: Center for Science in the Public Interest, 1999.

Jawad, A. S., and D. G. Scott. "Immunisation Triggering Rheumatoid Arthritis?" *Annals of the Rheumatic Diseases* 48, no. 2 (1989): 174. doi:10.1136/ard.48.2.174-a.

"Juvenile Arthritis." The Arthritis Foundation. Accessed December 10, 2010. http://www.arthritis.org/ja-daily-life.php.

Kobylewski, Sarah, PhD. Candidate, and Michael F. Jacobson, Ph.D. *Food Dyes A Rainbow of Risks*. Report. Washington, DC: Center for Science in the Public Interest, 2010.

"Late Effects of Treatment for Childhood Cancer (PDQ)." National Cancer Institute at the National Institutes of Health. Accessed August 27, 2012. http://cancer.gov/cancertopics/pdq/treatment/lateeffects/HealthProfessional.

"Learning Disability Fast Facts." National Center for Learning Disabilities. Accessed September 26, 2012. http://www.ncld.org/types-learning-disabilities/what-is-ld/learning-disability-fast-facts.

LeFever, Gretchen B., PhD, Andrea P. Arcona, and David O. Antonuccio. "ADHD among American Schoolchildren Evidence of Overdiagnosis and Overuse of Medication." *The Scientific Review of Mental Health Practice* 2, no. 1 (Spring/Summer 2003). http://www.srmhp.org/0201/adhd.html.

Lipman, T. H., Y. Chang, and K. M. Murphy. "The Epidemiology of Type 1 Diabetes in Children in Philadelphia 1990–1994: Evidence of an Epidemic." *Diabetes Care* 25, no. 11 (2002): 1969–975. doi:10.2337/diacare.25.11.1969.

Lipman, Terri H., PHD, CRNP, Lorraine E. Levitt Katz, MD, Sarah J. Ratcliffe, PhD, Kathryn M. Murphy, PHD, RN, Alexandra Aguilar, MD, Iraj Rezvani, MD, Carol J. Howe, MSN, RN, Shruti Fadia, MD, and Elizabeth Suarez, MD. "Increasing Incidence of Type 1 Diabetes in Youth, Twenty Years of the Philadelphia Pediatric Diabetes Registry." *Diabetes Care*, January 22, 2013. doi:10.2337/dc12-0767.

Luby, J. L., X. Si, A. C. Belden, M. Tandon, and E. Spitznagel. "Preschool Depression: Homotypic Continuity and Course Over 24 Months." *Archives of General Psychiatry* 66, no. 8 (2009): 897–905. doi:10.1001/archgenpsychiatry.2009.97.

Malaty, Hoda M., Xiaolin Fan, Antone R. Opekun, Carolyn Thibodeaux, and George D. Ferry. "Rising Incidence of Inflammatory Bowel Disease Among Children: A 12-year Study." *Journal of Pediatric Gastroenterology and Nutrition* 50, no. 1 (2010): 27–31. doi:10.1097/MPG.0b013e3181b99baa.

Mccann, D., A. Barrett, A. Cooper, D. Crumpler, L. Dalen, K. Grimshaw, E. Kitchin, K. Lok, L. Porteous, and E. Prince. "Food Additives and Hyperactive Behaviour in 3-year-old and 8/9-year-old Children in the Community: A Randomised, Double-blinded, Placebo-controlled Trial." *The Lancet* 370, no. 9598 (2007): 1560–567. doi:10.1016/S0140-6736(07)61306-3.

"Mercury-Human Exposure." U.S. Environmental Protection Agency. Accessed August 26, 2012. http://www.epa.gov/hg/exposure.htm.

M-M-R II (Measles, Mumps, and Rubella Virus Vaccine Live). Product insert. Merck and Co., Inc. Issued February 2006 and December 2007.

Moreno, C., MD, G. Laje, MD, C. Blanco, MD, PhD, H. Jiang, PhD, A. B. Schmidt, CSW, and M. Olfson, MD, MPH. "National Trends in the Outpatient Diagnosis and Treatment of Bipolar Disorder in Youth." *Archives of General Psychiatry* 64, no. 9 (September 01, 2007): 1032–039. doi:10.1001/archpsyc.64.9.1032.

Murray, Bob, PhD, and Alicia Fortinberry, MS. "Depression Fact Sheet: Depression Statistics and Depression Causes." Uplift Program. January 15, 2005. Accessed September 19, 2012. http://www.upliftprogram.com/depression_stats.html.

The National Academies. Office of News and Public Information. "Major Advances in Biology Should Be Used to Assess Birth Defects From Toxic Chemicals." News release, June 1, 2000. http://www8.nationalacademies.org/onpinews/newsitem.aspx?RecordID=9871.

"National Cancer Institute Factsheet—Childhood Cancers." National Cancer Institute at the National Institutes of Health. Accessed September 05, 2012. http://www.cancer.gov/cancertopics/factsheet/Sites-Types/childhood.

Newbold, R., E. Padillabanks, R. Snyder, T. Phillips, and W. Jefferson. "Developmental Exposure to Endocrine Disruptors and the Obesity Epidemic." *Reproductive Toxicology* 23, no. 3 (2007): 290–96. doi:10.1016/j.reprotox.2006.12.010.

Newmark, Sanford C. "Nutritional Intervention in ADHD." *EXPLORE: The Journal of Science and Healing* 5, no. 3 (May/June 2009): 171–74. doi:10.1016/j.explore.2009.03.006.

"Nutrition in the First 1,000 Days: State of the World's Mothers 2012." Save the Children. May 2012. Accessed August 29, 2012. http://www.savethechildren.org/atf/cf/%7B9def2ebe-10ae-432c-9bd0-df91d2eba74a%7D/STATE-OF-THE-WORLDS-MOTHERS-REPORT-2012-FINAL.PDF.

Panush, Richard S. "Food Induced ('Allergic') Arthritis: Clinical and Serological Studies." *The Journal of Rheumatology* 17, no. 3, 291–94.

Portuese, Enrico, and Trevor Orchard. "Mortality in Insulin-Dependent Diabetes." *Diabetes in America* 2 (1995): 221–232.

ProQuad. (Measles, Mumps, Rubella, and Varicella (OKA/Merck) Virus Vaccine Live. Product insert, Merck and Co., Inc. Issued July 2006.

Rajaratnam, Julie Knoll, Jake R. Marcus, Abraham D. Flaxman, Haidong Wang, Alison Levin-Rector, Laura Dwyer, Megan Costa, Alan D. Lopez, and Christopher JL Murray. "Neonatal, Postneonatal, Childhood, and Under-5 Mortality for 187 Countries, 1970–2010: A Systematic Analysis of Progress towards Millennium Development Goal 4." *The Lancet* 375, no. 9730 (2010): 1988–2008. doi:10.1016/S0140-6736(10)60703-9.

RECOMBIVAX HB (Hepatitis B Vaccine Recombinant). Product insert, Merck and Co., Inc. Accessed online at: https://www.merck.com/product/usa/pi_circulars/r/recombivax_hb/recombivax_pi.pd.

Rice, Catherine, PhD. "Prevalence of Autism Spectrum Disorders—Autism and Developmental Disabilities Monitoring Network, United States, 2006." *CDC Morbidity and Mortality Weekly Report (MMWR)* 58, no. SS10 (December 18, 2009): 1–20. http://www.cdc.gov/mmwr/preview/mmwrhtml/ss5810a1.htm.

"Second National Report on Human Exposure to Environmental Chemicals." Centers for Disease Control and Prevention. October 10, 2012. http://www.cdc.gov/exposurereport.

Sibilia, J., and J. Maillefert. "Vaccination and Rheumatoid Arthritis." *Annals of the Rheumatic Diseases* 61, no. 7 (July 2002): 575–76. doi:10.1136/ard.61.7.575.

Sicherer, Scott H., Anne Muñoz-Furlong, James H. Godbold, and Hugh A. Sampson. "US Prevalence of Self-reported Peanut, Tree Nut, and Sesame Allergy: 11-year Follow-up." *Journal of Allergy and Clinical Immunology* 125, no. 6 (2010): 1322–326. doi:10.1016/j.jaci.2010.03.029.

Smith, Jeffery. "Genetically Modified Foods . . . Are They Safe?" Institute of Responsible Technology. Accessed September 17, 2012. http://www.responsibletechnology.org/

The State of the World's Children 2015: Reimagine the Future: Innovation for Every Child. November 2014. Digital Report, UNICEF, 3 United Nations Plaza, New York, NY.

"Surviving the First Day: State of the World's Mothers 2012." Save the Children. May 2013. Accessed June 6, 2013. http://www.savethechildrenweb.org/SOWM-2013/.

"Understanding Obesogens." The Dr. Oz Show. Accessed September 28, 2010. http://www.doctoroz.com/videos/understanding-obesogens?page=2.

UNFPA, UNICEF, WHO, World Bank. "Trends in Maternal Mortality:1990–2010." UNFPA. 2012. Accessed September 12, 2012. http://www.unfpa.org/public/cache/offonce/home/publications/pid/10728;jsessionid=72E53FE857D0BD46635D58D57339F371.jahia02.

United States. Agency for Healthcare Research and Quality. *Attention-Deficit Hyperactivity Disorder (ADHD) in Children, Ages 5–17: Use and Expenditures, 2007 Statistical Brief*

#276. By Anita Soni, PhD. December 2009. http://meps.ahrq.gov/mepsweb/data_files/publications/st276/stat276.pdf.

United States. Agency for Healthcare Research and Quality. *Health Care Expenditures for the Five Most Common Children's Conditions, 2008: Estimates for U.S. Civilian Noninstitutionalized Children, Ages 0–17 | Statistical Brief #349.* By Marc Roemer, MS. December 2011. http://meps.ahrq.gov/mepsweb/data_files/publications/st349/stat349.pdf.

United States. Centers for Disease Control and Prevention. National Center for Health Statistics. *Infant Mortality Statistics from the 2013 Period Linked Birth/Infant Death Data Set.* By T. J. Matthews, Marian F. MacDorman, and Marie E. Thoma. Accessed December 12, 2015. http://www.cdc.gov/nchs/data/nvsr/nvsr64/nvsr64_09.pdf.

United States. Centers for Disease Control and Prevention. National Center for Health Statistics. *Prevalence of Obesity Among Children and Adolescents: United States, Trends 1963–1965 Through 2007–2008.* By Cynthia Ogden, PhD and Margaret Carroll, MSPH. Accessed April 28, 2010. http://www.cdc.gov/nchs/data/hestat/obesity_child_07_08/obesity_child_07_08.htm.

United States. Centers for Disease Control and Prevention. National Center for Health Statistics. *NCHS Fact Sheet: NCHS Data on Obesity.* February 2012. http://www.cdc.gov/nchs/data/factsheets/factsheet_obesity.htm.

United States. Centers for Disease Control and Prevention. National Center for Injury Prevention and Control. *Suicide—Facts at a Glance.* Summer 2010. Accessed September 18, 2012. http://www.cdc.gov/violenceprevention/pdf/Suicide_DataSheet-a.pdf.

United States. Centers for Disease Control and Prevention. National Center for Chronic Disease Prevention and Health Promotion. *Arthritis: Childhood Arthritis.* August 2011. http://www.cdc.gov/arthritis/basics/childhood.htm.

United States. Centers for Disease Control and Prevention. National Center Health Statistics. *NCHS Data Brief: Recent Trends in Infant Mortality in the United States.* By Marion F. MacDorman, PhD and T. J. Mathews, MS. October 2008. Accessed April 15, 2010. http://www.cdc.gov/nchs/data/databriefs/db09.pdf.

United States. Centers for Disease Control and Prevention. National Center Health Statistics. *NCHS Data Brief: Trends in Asthma Prevalence, Health Care Use, and Mortality in the United States, 2001–2010.* By Lara J. Akinbami, MD, Jeanne E. Moorman, MS, Cathy Bailey, MS, Hatice S. Zahran, MD, Michael King, PhD, Carol A. Johnson, MPH, and Xiang Liu, M.Sc. May 2012. www.cdc.gov/nchs/data/databriefs/db94.pdf.

United States. Centers for Disease Control and Prevention. NCHS. *Attention Deficit Hyperactivity Disorder Among Children Aged 5-17 Years in the United States, 1998-2009.* By Lara J. Akinbami, MD, Xiang Liu, MS, Patricia N. Pastor, PhD, and Cynthia A. Reuben, MA. August 11, 2011. http://www.cdc.gov/nchs/data/databriefs/db70.pdf.

United States. Centers for Disease Control and Prevention. National Center Health Statistics. *NCHS Data Brief Number 10 October 2008. Food Allergy among U.S. Children: Trends in Prevalence and Hospitalizations.* By Amy M. Branum, MSPH and Susan L. Lukacs, DO, MPH. Accessed September 17, 2012. http://www.cdc.gov/nchs/data/databriefs/db10.htm.

United States. Centers for Disease Control and Prevention. Office of Analysis and Epidemiology. *The State of Childhood Asthma, United States, 1980–2005.* By Lara J. Akinbami, MD. Vol. 381. Hyattsville, MD: NCHS, 2006.

United States. Centers for Disease Control and Prevention. Office of the Associate Director for Communication, Division of News and Electronic Media. *CDC Features: Estimates Childhood Arthritis National and State Estimates of Childhood Arthritis and Other Rheumatic Conditions.* July 06, 2010. http://www.cdc.gov/Features/dsPediatricArthritis/index.html.

United States. Centers for Disease Control and Prevention. Office of the Associate Director for Communication. *CDC Features: New Data on Autism Spectrum Disorders.* March 29, 2012. http://www.cdc.gov/features/countingautism/.

United States. Central Intelligence Agency. *Online World Factbook: Infant Mortality Country Comparison.* Accessed December 6, 2016. https://www.cia.gov/library/publications/the-world-factbook/rankorder/2091rank.html.

United States. Department of Health and Human Services. *Healthy People 2020, Mental Health.* Accessed September 18, 2012. http://www.healthypeople.gov/2020/LHI/mentalHealth.aspx.

United States. Department of Health and Human Services. National Cancer Institute. *Reducing Environmental Cancer Risk, What We Can Do Now—2008–2009 Annual Report President's Cancer Panel.* By Suzanne H. Reuben. April 2010. http://deainfo.nci.nih.gov/advisory/pcp/annualReports/pcp08-09rpt/PCP_Report_08-09_508.pdf.

United States. National Cancer Institute. Survellience, Epidemiology, and End Results Program. *SEER Cancer Statistics Review, 1975–2010.* By N. Howlader, A. M. Noone, M. Krapcho, J. Garshell, N. Neyman, S. F. Altekruse, C. L. Kosary, M. Yu, J. Ruhl, Z. Tatalovich, H. Cho, A. Mariotto, D. R. Lewis, H. S. Chen, E. J. Feuer, and K. A. Cronin. April 2013. http://seer.cancer.gov/csr/1975_2010/.

United States. National Institutes of Health. National Institute of Mental Health. *Depression in Children and Adolescents (Fact Sheet).* Accessed September 18, 2012. http://www.nimh.nih.gov/health/publications/depression-in-children-and-adolescents/index.shtml.

United States. National Institutes of Health. National Cancer Institute. *A Snapshot of Pediatric Cancers.* October 2011. Accessed August 29, 2012. http://www.cancer.gov/PublishedContent/Files/aboutnci/servingpeople/snapshots/2011_Pediatric_snapshot.508.pdf.

United States. Department of Education. National Center for Education Statistics. *The Condition of Education 2010, NCES 2010 - 028.* By Susan Aud, William Hussar, Michael Planty, Thomas Snyder, Kevin Bianco, Mary Ann Fox, Lauren Frohlich, Jana Kemp, and Lauren Drake. May 2010. http://nces.ed.gov/pubs2010/2010028.pdf.

United States. Department of Education. National Center for Education Statistics. *The Condition of Education 2012, NCES 2012-045.* By Susan Aud, William Hussar, Frank Johnson, Grace Kena, Erin Roth, Eileen Manning, Xiaolei Wang, and Jijun Zhang. May 2012. http://nces.ed.gov/pubs2012/2012045.pdf.

Van Cleave, J., S. L. Gortmaker, and J. M. Perrin. "Dynamics of Obesity and Chronic Health Conditions among Children and Youth." *JAMA: The Journal of the American Medical Association* 303, no. 7 (2010): 623–30. doi:10.1001/jama.2010.104.

Vehik, K., R. F. Hamman, D. Lezotte, J. M. Norris, G. Klingensmith, C. Bloch, M. Rewers, and D. Dabelea. "Increasing Incidence of Type 1 Diabetes in 0- to 17-Year-Old Colorado Youth." *Diabetes Care* 30, no. 3 (2007): 503–09. doi:10.2337/dc06-1837.

Visser, Susanna N., Melissa L. Danielson, Rebecca H. Bitsko, Joseph R. Holbrook, Michael D. Kogan, Reem M. Ghandour, Ruth Perou, and Stephen J. Blumberg. "Trends in the Parent-Report of Health Care Provider-Diagnosed and Medicated Attention-Deficit/Hyperactivity Disorder: United States, 2003–2011." *Journal of the American Academy of Child & Adolescent Psychiatry* 53, no. 1 (2014): 34–46.e2. doi:10.1016/j.jaac.2013.09.001.

Wall Street Journal. "Are ADHD Medications Overprescribed?" September 14, 2012. Accessed September 17, 2012. http://online.wsj.com/article/SB10000872396390444301704577631591596516110.html.

Weil, Elizabeth. "Puberty Before Age 10: A New 'Normal'?" *New York Times*, March 30, 2012. http://www.nytimes.com/2012/04/01/magazine/puberty-before-age-10-a-new-normal. html?pagewanted=2&_r=3.

Wilde Mathews, Anna. "So Young and So Many Pills." *Wall Street Journal*, December 28, 2010. http://online.wsj.com/article/SB10001424052970203731004576046073896475588.html.

Williams, Sarah C.P. "Gone Too Soon: What's Behind the High U.S. Infant Mortality Rate." *Stanford Medicine* Special Report (Fall 2012). Accessed March 21, 2016. http://sm.stanford. edu/archive/stanmed/2013fall/article2.html.

Windham, B., Ed. "Effects of Toxic Metals on Learning Ability and Behavior." Best Practice Assessment of Psychosis. February 23, 2012. http://psychoticdisorders.wordpress.com/ category/exposure-to-toxins/.

Woodruff, Tracey J., Daniel A. Axelrad, Amy D. Kyle, Onyemaechi Nweke, Gregory G. Miller, and Bradford J. Hurley. "Trends in Environmentally Related Childhood Illnesses." *Pediatrics* 113 (April 2004): 1133–140.

Worcester, S. "Childhood Arthritis Prevalence, Prognosis Eyed." *Pediatric News* 41, no. 6 (June 2007): 36. doi:10.1016/S0031-398X(07)70386-7.

Writing Group for the SEARCH for Diabetes in Youth Study Group, D. Dabelea, R. A. Bell, R. B. D'Agostino, Jr., G. Imperatore, J. M. Johansen, B. Linder, L. L. Liu, B. Loots, S. Marcovina, E. J. Mayer-Davis, D. J. Pettitt, and B. Waitzfelder. "Incidence of Diabetes in Youth in the United States." *JAMA: The Journal of the American Medical Association* 297, no. 24 (June 27, 2007): 2716–724. doi:10.1001/jama.297.24.2716.

Zarcone, Dana. "The Alarming Statistics on Childhood Depression." Ezine Articles. Accessed September 18, 2012. http://ezinearticles.com/?The-Alarming-Statistics-on-Childhood-Depression&id=4877622.

Zuvekas, S. H., and B. Vitiello. "Stimulant Medication Use in Children: A 12-year Perspective." *American Journal of Psychiatry* 169, no. 2 (February 2012): 160–66. http://www.ncbi.nlm. nih.gov/pubmed/22420039.

Chapter 4

Grossman, Elizabeth. "Banned in Europe, Safe in the U.S." Ensia. June 09, 2014. http://ensia. com/features/banned-in-europe-safe-in-the-u-s/.

HCCI. "Press Release: Children's Health Care Spending Report 2007–2010." News release, July 1, 2012. Health Care Cost Institute. Accessed September 18, 2012. http://www. healthcostinstitute.org/news-and-events/press-release-childrens-health-care-spending-report-2007-2010.

"How People Are Exposed to Mercury." U.S. Environmental Protection Agency. Accessed September 05, 2012. http://www.epa.gov/hg/exposure.htm.

"Mercury - Human Exposure." U.S. Environmental Protection Agency. Accessed August 26, 2012. http://www.epa.gov/hg/exposure.htm

"Mercury Compounds Hazard Summary." U.S. Environmental Protection Agency. Accessed May 11, 2015. http://www.epa.gov/ttn/atw/hlthef/mercury.html.

"Minimal Risk Levels (MRLs) for Hazardous Substances." Agency for Toxic Substances and Disease Registry (ATSDR). Accessed May 05, 2015. http://www.atsdr.cdc.gov/mrls/mrllist. asp#24tag.

"Thimerosal in Vaccines Questions and Answers." U.S. Food and Drug Administration. Accessed September 05, 2012. http://www.fda.gov/BiologicsBloodVaccines/Vaccines/ QuestionsaboutVaccines/ucm070430.htm.

U.S. Environmental Protection Agency. "FDA and EPA Issue Updated Draft Advice for Fish Consumption/ Advice Encourages Pregnant Women and Breastfeeding Mothers to Eat

More Fish That Are Lower in Mercury." News release, June 09, 2014. U.S. Environmental Protection Agency. http://yosemite.epa.gov/opa/admpress.nsf/Press%20Releases%20 from%20Headquarters?OpenView.

United States. Agency for Healthcare Research and Quality. *Health Care Expenditures for the Five Most Common Children's Conditions, 2008: Estimates for U.S. Civilian Noninstitutionalized Children, Ages 0-17 Statistical Brief #349.* By Marc Roemer, MS. December 2011. http:// meps.ahrq.gov/mepsweb/data_files/publications/st349/stat349.pdf.

United States. Department of Health and Human Services. National Cancer Institute. *Reducing Environmental Cancer Risk, What We Can Do Now—2008–2009 Annual Report President's Cancer Panel.* By Suzanne H. Reuben. April 2010. http://deainfo.nci.nih.gov/advisory/pcp/ annualReports/pcp08-09rpt/PCP_Report_08-09_508.pdf.

Chapter 5

"Adoption of Genetically Engineered Crops in the U.S." United States Department of Agriculture Economic Research Service. July 14, 2014. http://www.ers.usda.gov/data-products/adoption-of-genetically-engineered-crops-in-the-us.aspx. http://www.easybib.com/ cite/view

"Animal Feed." GRACE Communications Foundation. Accessed February 20, 2013. http:// www.sustainabletable.org/260/animal-feed.

"AquAdvantage Salmon." U.S. Food and Drug Administration. Accessed November 19, 2015. http://www.fda.gov/AnimalVeterinary/DevelopmentApprovalProcess/GeneticEngineering/ GeneticallyEngineeredAnimals/ucm280853.htm.

"Aquafarming." PETA. Accessed May 20, 2013. http://www.peta.org/issues/animals-used-for-food/aquafarming.aspx.

Aris, Aziz, and Samuel Leblanc. "Maternal and Fetal Exposure to Pesticides Associated to Genetically Modified Foods in Eastern Townships of Quebec, Canada." *Reproductive Toxicology* 31, no. 4 (2011): 528–33. doi:10.1016/j.reprotox.2011.02.004.

Artificial Colors. Feingold Association of the United States. Accessed September 19, 2012. http:// www.feingold.org/Research/BLUE/Page-06-7-colorsBHT.pdf.

"Background on the FDA Food Safety Modernization Act (FSMA)." FDA. Accessed April 18, 2013. http://www.fda.gov/NewsEvents/PublicHealthFocus/ucm239907.htm.

Barry, Ellen. "Russia Announces Barriers on Imports of U.S. Meat." *New York Times*, December 8, 2012. http://www.nytimes.com/2012/12/09/world/europe/russia-announces-barriers-on-imports-of-us-meat.html?_r=1&.

Baumann, Jeremiah, Julie Wolk, Jane Houlihan, and Richard Wiles. *Brain Food—What Women Should Know about Mercury Contamination of Fish.* Report. Washington, D.C.: Environmental Working Group, 2001. http://static.ewg.org/reports/2001/BrainFood.pdf.

Bean, Nancy H., PhD, Joy S. Goulding, Christopher Lao, and Frederick J. Angulo, DVM, PhD. "Surveillance for Foodborne-Disease Outbreaks—United States, 1988–1992." *CDC Morbidity and Mortality Weekly Report (MMWR)* 45, no. SS-5 (October 25, 1996): 1–55. http://www.cdc.gov/mmwr/preview/mmwrhtml/00044241.htm.

"Bioengineered Food: Statement of James Maryanski, FDA Biotechnology Coordinator, Before the Senate Committee on Agriculture, Nutrition and Forestry, October 7, 1999." U.S. Food and Drug Administration. Accessed February 18, 2015. http://www.fda.gov/NewsEvents/ Testimony/ucm115040.htm.

Bolan, N. S., A. A. Szogi, T. Chuasavathi, B. Seshadri, M. J. Rothrock, and P. Panneerselvam. "Uses and Management of Poultry Litter." *World's Poultry Science Journal* 66, no. 04 (2010): 673–98. doi:10.1017/S0043933910000656.

Calton, Jayson, Mira Calton, and Mark Sisson. *Rich Food Poor Food: The Ultimate Grocery Purchasing System (GPS)*. Malibu, CA: Primal Blueprint Pub., 2013.

Centers for Disease Control and Prevention. Accessed December 29, 2016. https://www.cdc.gov/foodborneburden/2011-foodborne-estimates.html

Center for Food Safety. "EPA Approves New 2, 4-D Herbicide Blend, Paving Way for Controversial GE Crops." News release, October 15, 2014. http://www.centerforfoodsafety.org/press-releases/3536/epa-app roves-new-24-d- herbicide-blend-paving-way-for-controversial-ge-crops.

"The Chicken Industry." PETA. Accessed May 15, 2013. http://www.peta.org/issues/animals-used-for-food/factory-farming/chickens/chicken-industry/. organic chicken immobile:

"Chicken Production on Factory Farms." Farmsanctuary. Accessed May 17, 2013. http://www.farmsanctuary.org/learn/factory-farming/chickens-used-for-meat/#.

Dean, Amy, DO, and Armstrong, Jennifer, MD. "Genetically Modified Foods Position Paper: The American Academy of Environmental Medicine (AAEM)." June 08, 2009. Accessed October 20, 2014. https://www.aaemonline.org/gmo.php.

Dennis, Brady. "FDA Finalizes Voluntary Rules on Phasing Out Certain Antibiotics in Livestock." *Washington Post*, December 11, 2013. http://www.washingtonpost.com/national/health-science/fda-finalizes-voluntary-rules-on-phasing-out-certain-antibiotics-in-livestock/2013/12/11/e64ca05c-61e8-11e3-8beb-3f9a9942850f_story.html.

Dona, A., and I. S. Arvanitoyannis. "Health Risk of Genetically Modified Foods." *Critical Reviews in Food Science and Nutrition 49, no. 2* (February 2009): 164–175. doi:10.1080/10408390701855993.

Dufault, Renee, Blaise Leblanc, Roseanne Schnoll, Charles Cornett, Laura Schweitzer, David Wallinga, Jane Hightower, Lyn Patrick, and Walter J. Lukiw. "Mercury from Chlor-alkali Plants: Measured Concentrations in Food Product Sugar." *Environmental Health* 8, no. 2 (January 2009): 2–7. doi:10.1186/1476-069X-8-2.

Eisler, Peter. "Growing Concern over Marketing Tainted Beef." *USA Today*, April 15, 2010. http://usatoday30.usatoday.com/news/washington/2010-04-12-tainted-meat_N.htm.

Emanuele, Patricia. "Antibiotic Resistance." *American Association of Occupational Health Nurses Journal* 58, no. 9 (2010): 363–65. doi:10.3928/08910162-20100826-03.

"Euro MPs Back Pesticide Controls." *BBC News*, January 13, 2009. http://news.bbc.co.uk/2/hi/uk_news/7825552.stm.

EWG Farm Subsidy Database. Accessed May 06, 2013. http://farm.ewg.org/progdetail.php?fips=00000&progcode=totalfarm&page=concionname=theUnitedStates.

"Factory Farming - Chickens on the Factory Farm." The Massachusetts Society for the Prevention of Cruelty to Animals—Angell Animal Medical Center. Accessed May 17, 2013. http://www.mspca.org/programs/animal-protection-legislation/animal-welfare/farm-animal-welfare/factory-farming/chicken/chickens-on-the-factory-farm.html.

"Factory Fish Farming." Food & Water Watch. Accessed May 20, 2013. http://www.foodandwaterwatch.org/fish/fish-farming/.

Fagan, John, Michael Antonio, and Claire Robinson. *GMO Myths and Truths. An Evidence-based Examination of GMO Claims (Second Edition)*. Report. London: Earth Open Source, 2012. Accessed May 20, 2015. http://earthopensource.org/wp-content/uploads/2014/11/GMO-Myths-and-Truths-edition2.pdf.

Fiengold Association of the United States. Colors, Flavors, BHT, Etc. Accessed November 17, 2013. http://www.feingold.org/Research/BLUE/Page-06-7-colorsBHT.pdf.

Finamore, Alberto, Marianna Roselli, Serena Britti, Giovanni Monastra, Roberto Ambra, Aida Turrini, and Elena Mengheri. "Intestinal and Peripheral Immune Response to MON810

Maize Ingestion in Weaning and Old Mice." *Journal of Agricultural and Food Chemistry J. Agric. Food Chem.* 56, no. 23 (2008): 11533-1539. doi:10.1021/jf802059w.

"Fish." Food & Water Watch. Accessed April 14, 2013. http://www.foodandwaterwatch.org/common-resources/fish/.

"Food Economics." GRACE Communications Foundation. Accessed May 14, 2013. http://www.sustainabletable.org/491/food-economics.

Food Inc. Directed by Robert Kenner. By Elise Pearlstein and Kim Roberts. Narrated by Michael Pollan and Eric Schlosser. Participant Media, 2008. Documentary.

Freese, William, and David Schubert. "*Safety Testing and Regulation of Genetically Engineered Foods.*" Biotechnology and Genetic Engineering Reviews 21, no. 1 (2004): 299–324. doi:10.1080/02648725.2004.10648060.

FSIS/USDA. "Recalled Beef." E-mail message to author, Joanne Stanton. January 11, 2013.

Garina, Anastasia. "Russia Throws Poisonous Meat Back to US." English Pravda.ru. December 11, 2012. http://english.pravda.ru/business/companies/11-12-2012/123129-russia_usa_meat_imports-0/.

"General Information Related to Microbiological Risks in Food." World Health Organization. Accessed April 17, 2013. http://www.who.int/foodsafety/micro/general/en/index.html.

"The GE Process." The Institute for Responsible Technology. Accessed May 15, 2013. http://www.responsibletechnology.org/GMO-BASICS/THE-GE-PROCESS.

Glyphosate; Pesticide Tolerance, 40 CFR 180 § 76 FR 27268 (2011). https://federalregister.gov/a/2011-11205

"GMOs FAQs." LabelGMOs. Accessed November 17, 2013. http://www.labelgmos.org/faqs.

"GMOs in Food." The Institute for Responsible Technology. Accessed May 12, 2013. http://www.responsibletechnology.org/gmo-basics/gmos-in-food.

Hyman, Mark, MD. "The Not-So-Sweet Truth About High Fructose Corn Syrup." The Huffington Post. May 16, 2011. http://www.huffingtonpost.com/dr-mark-hyman/high-fructose-corn-syrup-dangers_b_861913.html?view=print&comm_ref=false.

"Industrial Agriculture." Union of Concerned Scientists. Accessed April 22, 2013. http://www.ucsusa.org/food_and_agriculture/our-failing-food-system/industrial-agriculture/they-eat-what-the-reality-of.html.

Jacobson, Michael F., PhD, and David Schardt, MS. *Diet, ADHD and Behavior: A Quarter Century of Review*. Report. Washington, DC: Center for Science in the Public Interest, 1999.

Jacobson, Mike. "Rainbow of Risks: Dye Graph Permission." E-mail message to author, Joanne Stanton. April 10, 2013.

"Key FDA Documents Revealing Hazards of Genetically Engineered Foods—and Flaws with How the Agency Made Its Policy." Alliance for Bio-Integrity. Accessed April 06, 2015. http://www.biointegrity.org/FDAdocs/04/view1.html.

Kılıç, Aysun, and M. Turan Akay. "A Three Generation Study with Genetically Modified Bt Corn in Rats: Biochemical and Histopathological Investigation." *Food and Chemical Toxicology* 46, no. 3 (2008): 1164–170. doi:10.1016/j.fct.2007.11.016.

Knowles, Toby G., Steve C. Kestin, Susan M. Haslam, Steven N. Brown, Laura E. Green, Andrew Butterworth, Stuart J. Pope, Dirk Pfeiffer, and Christine J. Nicol. "Leg Disorders in Broiler Chickens: Prevalence, Risk Factors and Prevention." Edited by Patrick Callaerts. *PLoS ONE* 3, no. 2 (2008): E1545. doi:10.1371/journal.pone.0001545.

Kobylewski, Sarah, PhD Candidate, and Michael F. Jacobson, PhD. *Food Dyes A Rainbow of Risks*. Report. Washington, DC: Center for Science in the Public Interest, 2010.

Kristof, Nicholas D. "Arsenic in Our Chicken?" *New York Times*, April 4, 2012. http://www.nytimes.com/2012/04/05/opinion/kristof-arsenic-in-our-chicken.html?_r=0.

Lepisto, Christine. "7 Foods Banned in Europe Still Available in the U.S." Care2. February 28, 2010. http://www.care2.com/greenliving/7-foods-banned-in-europe-still-available-in-the-us.html.

"Major Crops Grown in the United States." U.S. Environmental Protection Agency. Accessed April 10, 2015. http://www.epa.gov/agriculture/ag101/cropmajor.html.

Mccann, D., A. Barrett, A. Cooper, D. Crumpler, L. Dalen, K. Grimshaw, E. Kitchin, K. Lok, L. Porteous, and E. Prince. "Food Additives and Hyperactive Behaviour in 3-year-old and 8/9-year-old Children in the Community: A Randomised, Double-blinded, Placebo-controlled Trial." *The Lancet* 370, no. 9598 (2007): 1560–567. doi:10.1016/S0140-6736(07)61306-3.

The Meatrix II: Revolting. Free Range Studio and Sustainable Table, 2006. Accessed June 01, 2015. www.themeatrix.com.

The Meatrix. Free Range Studio and Sustainable Table, 2006. Accessed June 01, 2015. www.themeatrix.com.

Mott, Lawrie, David Fore, Jennifer Curtis, and Gina Solomon. *Our Children At Risk: The Five Worst Environmental Threats to Their Health. Chapter 5 Pesticides.* Report. New York: Natural Resources Defense Council Publication, 1997. Accessed April 02, 2015. http://www.nrdc.org/health/kids/ocar/chap5.asp.

"Myths & Realities of GE Crops." Center for Food Safety. Accessed February 18, 2015. http://www.centerforfoodsafety.org/issues/311/ge-foods/myths-and-realities-of-ge-crops.

Nachman, Keeve E., Patrick A. Baron, Georg Raber, Kevin A. Francesconi, Ana Navas-Acien, and David C. Love. "Roxarsone, Inorganic Arsenic, and Other Arsenic Species in Chicken: A U.S.-Based Market Basket Sample." *Environmental Health Perspectives* 121, no. 7 (2013): 818–24. doi:10.1289/ehp.1206245.

Nsouli, T. M., S. M. Nsouli, R. E. Linde, F. O'Mara, R. T. Scanlon, and J. A. Bellanti. "Role of Food Allergy in Serious Otitis Media." *Annals of Allergy* 73, no. 3 (September 1994): 215–19.

Paul, Katherine, and Ronnie Cummins, eds. "GMO Salmon Would Be Approved as 'New Animal Drug'." *Organic Bytes #361*, January 2013. http://www.organicconsumers.org/bytes/ob361.htm.

Pesticide Action Network UK / A Catalogue of Lists of Pesticides Identifying Those Associated with Particularly Harmful or Environmental Impacts. Publication. 2009. http://www.pan-europe.info/Campaigns/pesticides/documents/cut_off/list%20of%20lists.pdf.

"Plunkett Research, Ltd." Food Beverage Grocery Market Research. Accessed December 05, 2013. http://www.plunkettresearch.com/food-beverage-grocery-market-research/industry-and-business-data.

Pollan, Michael. "Farmer In Chief." New York Times. October 11, 2008. http://www.nytimes.com/2008/10/12/magazine/12policy-t.html?pagewanted=all.

"Poverty Threatens Health of US Children." ScienceDaily. March 4, 2013. http://www.sciencedaily.com/releases/2013/05/130504163257.htm.

"Public Sentiment about Genetically Modified Food." Http://www.pewtrusts.org/uploadedFiles/wwwpewtrustsorg/Public_Opinion/Food_and_Biotechnology/survey3-01.pdf. Accessed November 15, 2013.

"Questions and Answers Regarding 3-Nitro (Roxarsone)." FDA - Animal & Veterinary. Accessed May 18, 2013. http://www.fda.gov/AnimalVeterinary/SafetyHealth/ProductSafetyInformation/ucm258313.htm.

Scallan, Elaine, Patricia M. Griffin, Frederick J. Angulo, Robert V. Tauxe, and Robert M. Hoekstra. "Foodborne Illness Acquired in the United States—Unspecified Agents." *Emerging Infectious Diseases* 17, no. 1 (January 2011). doi:10.3201/eid1701.P21101.

"Seafood." GRACE Communications Foundation. Accessed May 20, 2013. http://www.gracelinks.org/898/seafood#fishfarming.

Seidler, Ramon J. "Pesticide Use on Genetically Engineered Crops." *Environmental Working Group Ag/Mag*, September 2014. Accessed April 02, 2015. http://static.ewg.org/agmag/pdfs/pesticide_use_on_genetically_engineered_crops.pdf.

Seidler, Ramon J., and David Bronner. "Traditional Soil-Applied Insecticides Are Surging Alongside Systemic Neonicotinoid Insecticides on Genetically Engineered Corn." (Addendum to "Pesticide Use on Genetically Engineered Crops") *Environmental Working Group Ag/Mag*, October 2015. Accessed March 02, 2015. http://static.ewg.org/agmag/pdfs/pesticide_use_on_genetically_engineered_crops.pdf.

Shiva, Vandana, Debbie Barker, and Caroline Lockhart. *The GMO Emperor Has No Clothes, A Global Citizens Report on the State of GMOs—False Promises, Failed Technologies*. Report. Accessed March 10, 2013. http://www.navdanyainternational.it/images/doc/Full_Report_Rapporto_completo.pdf.

Smith, Jeffrey M. Genetic Roulette: *The Documented Health Risks of Genetically Engineered Foods*. Fairfield, IA: Yes! Books, 2007.

Smith, Jeffrey. "State of the Science on the Health Risks of GM Food." Institute of Responsible Technology. 2013. Accessed May 15, 2015. http://responsibletechnology.org/State-of-Science-Health-Risks.pdf.

Sorensen, Janelle. "Why Did the Chicken Take a Bath in Chlorine?" *WebMD* (blog), March 7, 2011. http://blogs.webmd.com/health-ehome/2011/03/why-did-the-chicken-take-a-bath-in-chlorine.html.

Sullivan, Preston. *Sustainable Corn and Soybean Production*. Publication. Fayetteville, Arkansas: National Center for Appropriate Technology, 2003.

"Sustainable Agriculture —The Basics." GRACE Communications Foundation. Accessed February 20, 2014. http://www.sustainabletable.org/246/sustainable-agriculture-the-basics.

"Sustainable Crop Production." GRACE Communications Foundation. Accessed May 22, 2013. http://gracelinks.org/249/sustainable-crop-production.http://www.gracelinks.org/253/organic-agriculture

"Sustainable Livestock Husbandry." GRACE Communications Foundation. Accessed May 22, 2013. http://www.gracelinks.org/248/sustainable-livestock-husbandry.

"U.S. Meat Production." Physicians for Social Responsiblity. Accessed May 21, 2013. http://www.psr.org/chapters/oregon/safe-food/industrial-meat-system.html.

"U.S. Polls on GE Food Labeling." Center for Food Safety. Accessed November 15, 2013. http://www.centerforfoodsafety.org/issues/976/ge-food-labeling/us-polls-on-ge-food-labeling.

Undurraga, Dawn. "PEW: FDA Allows Untested Chemicals in Food." Evironmental Working Group. August 14, 2014. http://www.ewg.org/enviroblog/2013/08/pew-analysis-finds-fda-allows-untested-chemicals-food.

United States. U.S. Department of Agriculture. National Organic Program. *USDA Agricultural Marketing Service*. By Linda Coffey and Ann H. Baier. November 2012. http://www.ams.usda.gov/AMSv1.0/getfile?dDocName=STELPRDC5101543.

United States. U.S. Department of Agriculture. Office of Inspector General. *FSIS National Residue Program for Cattle*. By Gil H. Harden. Washington, D.C., 2010. http://www.usda.gov/oig/webdocs/24601-08-KC.pdf. Audit Report 24601-08-KC

United States. U.S. Department of Agriculture. AIB: Agricultural Information Bulletin. *The Seed Industry in U.S. Agriculture: An Exploration of Data and Information on Crop Seed Markets, Regulation, Industry Structure, and Research and Development*. By Jorge Fernandez-Cornejo. February 2004. http://www.ers.usda.gov/publications/aib-agricultural-information-bulletin/aib786.aspx#.U2lJLqLYDLQ.

United States. U.S. Department of Agriculture. Economic Research Service. *USDA ERS - Adoption of Genetically Engineered Crops in the U.S.: Recent Trends in GE Adoption.* Accessed May 03, 2015.http://www.ers.usda.gov/data-products/adoption-of-genetically-engineered-crops-in-the-us/recent-trends-in-ge-adoption.aspx#.VDrS2Pn.

Vendômois, Joël Spiroux De. "A Comparison of the Effects of Three GM Corn Varieties on Mammalian Health." *International Journal of Biological Sciences Int. J. Biol. Sci.*, 2009, 706–26. doi:10.7150/ijbs.5.706.

Verma, Charu, Surabhi Nanda, R. K. Singh, R. B. Singh, and Sanjay Mishra. "A Review on Impacts of Genetically Modified Food on Human Health." *The Open Nutraceuticals Journal* 4, no. 1 (2011): 3–11. doi:10.2174/1876396001104010003.

"Victories." Farm Forward. Accessed May 15, 2013. http://www.farmforward.com/farming-forward/victories.

"Whole Foods Market GMO Labeling Announcement Reverberating Through Industry." Institute for Responsible Technology. Accessed May 12, 2013. http://www.responsibletechnology.org/posts/whole-foods-market-gmo-labeling-announcement-reverberating-through-industry/.

World Health Organization. The International Agency for Research on Cancer. "IARC Monographs Volume 112: Evaluation of Five Organophosphate Insecticides and Herbicides." News release, March 20, 2015. Accessed May 01, 2015. http://www.iarc.fr/en/media-centre/iarcnews/pdf/MonographVolume112.pdf.

Chapter 6

21 Code of Federal Regulation, 4 § 201.323 (2013).

21 Code of Federal Regulation, 7 § 610.15 (2014).

"Aluminum in Vaccines: What You Should Know." *Q&A: Vaccine Education Center at The Children's Hospital of Philadelphia* 5 (Winter 2014). http://vec.chop.edu/export/download/pdfs/articles/vaccine-education-center/aluminum.pdf.

"Are Too Many Kids Taking Antipsychotic Drugs? Use Is Climbing despite Questions about How Safe the Drugs Are and How Well They Work." *Consumer Reports*, December 2013. http://www.consumerreports.org/cro/2013/12/are-too-many-kids-taking-antipsychotic-drugs/index.htm.

Bishop, Nicholas J., Ruth Morley, J. Philip Day, and Alan Lucas. "Aluminum Neurotoxicity in Preterm Infants Receiving Intravenous-Feeding Solutions." *New England Journal of Medicine* 336, no. 22 (1997): 1557–562. doi:10.1056/nejm199705293362203.

"Boost Your Child's Immune System." Ask Dr Sears, the Trusted Resource for Parents. August 30, 2013. Accessed March 5, 2015. http://www.askdrsears.com/topics/health-concerns/vaccines/boost-childs-immune-system.

Bruesewitz V. Wyeth LLC, No. 09-152 (February 22, 2011), 2010 Term Opinions, 15.

"Cancer, Simian Virus 40 (SV40), and Polio Vaccine Fact Sheet." Centers for Disease Control and Prevention. Accessed December 2, 2013. http://web.archive.org/web/20130522091608/http://www.cdc.gov/vaccinesafety/updates/archive/polio_and_cancer_factsheet.htm.

"CDC Publishes First National Study on Use of Behavioral Therapy, Medication, and Dietary Supplements for ADHD in Children." Centers for Disease Control and Prevention. April 01, 2015. Accessed April 15, 2015. http://www.cdc.gov/media/releases/2015/p0401-adhd.html.

Chamey, P. "A.S.P.E.N. Statement on Aluminum in Parenteral Nutrition Solutions." *Nutrition in Clinical Practice* 19, no. 4 (2004): 416–17. doi:10.1177/0115426504019004416.

The Childhood Immunization Schedule and Safety: Stakeholder Concerns, Scientific Evidence, and Future Studies. Washington, D.C.: National Academies Press, 2013. Accessed February 1, 2015. http://www.iom.edu/Reports/2013/The-Childhood-Immunization-Schedule-and-Safety.aspx.

Chung, Eun Hee. "Vaccine Allergies." *Clinical and Experimental Vaccine Research* 3, no. 1 (January 2014): 50–57. doi:10.7774/cevr.2014.3.1.50.

Classen, J. Barthelow. "Review of Vaccine Induced Immune Overload and the Resulting Epidemics of Type 1 Diabetes and Metabolic Syndrome, Emphasis on Explaining the Recent Accelerations in the Risk of Prediabetes and Other Immune Mediated Diseases." *Journal of Molecular and Genetic Medicine* 02, no. S1 (2014). Accessed March 10, 2015. doi:10.4172/1747-0862.s1-025.

Coeytaux, Fancine, Debra Bingham, and Nan Strauss. "Maternal Mortality in the United States: A Human Rights Failure." *Contraception Editorial*, March 2011, 189–93. Accessed September 17, 2012. http://www.arhp.org/publications-and-resources/contraception-journal/march-2011.

Comer, Jonathan S., Mark Olfson, and Ramin Mojtabai. "National Trends in Child and Adolescent Psychotropic Polypharmacy in Office-Based Practice, 1996–2007." *Journal of the American Academy of Child & Adolescent Psychiatry* 49, no. 10 (2010): 1001–010. doi:10.1016/j.jaac.2010.07.007.

"Common Ingredients in U.S. Licensed Vaccines." U.S. Food and Drug Administration. Accessed May 30, 2014. http://www.fda.gov/BiologicsBloodVaccines/SafetyAvailability/VaccineSafety/ucm187810.htm.

"Current VISs." Centers for Disease Control and Prevention. October 22, 2014. Accessed November 14, 2014. http://www.cdc.gov/vaccines/hcp/vis/current-vis.html.

DeStefano, Frank, Tanya Karapurkar Bhasin, William W. Thompson, Marshalyn Yeargin-Allsopp, and Coleen Boyle. "Age at First Measles-Mumps-Rubella Vaccination in Children with Autism and School-matched Control Subjects: A Population-Based Study in Metropolitan Atlanta." *Pediatrics* 113, no. 2 (February 01, 2004): 259–66. Accessed September 01, 2015. doi:10.1542/peds.113.2.259.

Diller, Lawrence H., MD. "Kids on Drugs—A Behavioral Pediatrician Questions the Wisdom of Medicating Our Children." Salon Media Group. March 9, 2000. Accessed February 21, 2014. http://www.salon.com/health/feature/2000/03/09/kid_drugs/index.html.

"Diphtheria, Tetanus, and Pertussis (DTaP) VIS." Centers for Disease Control and Prevention. Accessed May 17, 2007. http://www.cdc.gov/vaccines/hcp/vis/vis-statements/dtap.html.

Dube, Nicole. *OLR Research Report: Mercury-Free Vaccine Legislation in Other States*. Report no. 2010-R-0352. Hartford: Connecticut General Assembly, 2010. Accessed June 05, 2015. http://www.cga.ct.gov/2010/rpt/2010-R-0352.htm.

"Early Estimates of Seasonal Influenza Vaccine Effectiveness." *Morbidity and Mortality Weekly Report* 64, no. 01 (January 16, 2015): 10–15. http://www.cdc.gov/mmwr/preview/mmwrhtml/mm6401a4.htm?s_cid=mm6401a4_e.

Eickhoff, T. C., and M. Myers. "Conference Report Workshop Summary Aluminum in Vaccines." *Vaccine* 20 (2002): S1–S4. http://archive.hhs.gov/nvpo/nvac/documents/Aluminumws.pdf.

El-Rahman, S. "Neuropathology of Aluminum Toxicity in Rats (glutamate and GABA Impairment)." *Pharmacological Research* 47, no. 3 (2003): 189–94. doi:10.1016/s1043-6618(02)00336-5.

Fallon, L. "Encephalitis Gale Encyclopedia of Children's Health: Infancy through Adolescence." Encyclopedia.com. 2006. Accessed February 25, 2015. http://www.encyclopedia.com/topic/encephalitis.aspx#1-1G2:3447200213-full.

Feeley, Jef, and Margaret Cronin Fisk. "J&J Hid Risks Risperdal Makes Boys' Breasts Grow: Lawyer." Bloomberg.com. September 24, 2012. http://www.bloomberg.com/news/2012-09-24/j-j-hid-risks-risperdal-makes-boys-breasts-grow-lawyer.html.

"Frequently Asked Questions about Adjuvants." Centers for Disease Control and Prevention. February 18, 2015. http://www.cdc.gov/vaccinesafety/concerns/adjuvants.html.

Gorman, Christine. "When the Vaccine Causes the Polio." *Time Magazine* 30 Oct. 1995: Vol. 146. No. 18. Pg. 83. Print.

Greenlee, John E., MD. "Encephalitis." Merck Manual Consumer Version. 2013. Accessed February 25, 2015. http://www.merckmanuals.com/home/brain_spinal_cord_and_nerve_disorders/brain_infections/encephalitis.html.

Halsey, N. A., and L. Goldman. "Balancing Risks and Benefits: Primum Non Nocere Is Too Simplistic." *Pediatrics* 108, no. 2 (2001): 466–67. doi:10.1542/peds.108.2.466.

Harris, Gardiner. "Advisers on Vaccines Often Have Conflicts, Report Says." *New York Times*, December 17, 2009. http://www.nytimes.com/2009/12/18/health/policy/18cdc.html?_r=0.

Ho, Beng-Choon, Nancy C. Andreasen, Steven Ziebell, Ronald Pierson, and Vincent Magnotta. "Long-tem Antipsychotic Treatment and Brain Volumes: A Longitudinal Study of First-Episode Schizophrenia." *Archives of General Psychology* 68, no. 2 (2011): 128–37. doi:10.1001/archgenpsychiatry.2010.199.

Holland, Mary, Louis Conte, Robert Krakow, and Lisa Colin. "Unanswered Questions from the Vaccine Injury Compensation Program: A Review of Compensated Cases of Vaccine-Induced Brain Injury." *Pace Environmental Law Review* 28, no. 2 (2011). http://digitalcommons.pace.edu/pelr/vol28/iss2/6.

"How Do Drugs and Biologics Differ?" Biotechnology Industry Organization. November 10, 2010. https://www.bio.org/articles/how-do-drugs-and-biologics-differ.

"Immunization Schedules. 1983 and 2015" Centers for Disease Control and Prevention. Accessed January 20, 2015. http://www.cdc.gov/vaccines/schedules/hcp/child-adolescent.html.

"IOWA Thimerosal Law." *Immunization Update: The Immunization Program Newsletter.* 1 (April 2006): 3. Accessed June 9, 2015. https://www.idph.state.ia.us/adper/common/pdf/immunization/newsletter/april_2006.pdf.

"Johnson & Johnson to Pay More Than $2.2 Billion to Resolve Criminal and Civil Investigations." Department of Justice. November 4, 2014. http://www.justice.gov/opa/pr/2013/November/13-ag-1170.html.

Kassebaum, Nicholas J., et al. "Global, Regional, and National Levels and Causes of Maternal Mortality during 1990–2013: A Systematic Analysis for the Global Burden of Disease Study 2013." *The Lancet* 384, no. 9947 (May 2, 2014): 980–1004. doi:10.1016/S0140-6736(14)60696-6.

Kessler, D. A. "Introducing MEDWatch. A New Approach to Reporting Medication and Device Adverse Effects and Product Problems." *JAMA: The Journal of the American Medical Association* 269, no. 21 (1993): 2765–768. doi:10.1001/jama.269.21.2765.

Klish, William J., MD, Susan S. Baker, MD, Carlos A. Flores, MD, Hael K. Georgieff, MD, Alan M. Lake, MD, Udolph L. Leibel, MD, and John N. Udall, Jr, MD, PhD. "Aluminum Toxicity in Infants and Children." *Pediatrics* 97 (1996): 413–16.

Lenzer, Jeanne. "Centers for Disease Control and Prevention: Protecting the Private Good?" *BMJ* 350, h2362. May 15, 2015. Accessed May 12, 2016. doi:10.1136/bmj.h2362.

Levin, Myron. "'91 Memo Warned of Mercury in Shots." *Latimes.com*, February 5, 2005. http://whale.to/vaccines/2005-02-08-LA-Times-1991-Memo-Warned-of-Mercury-in-Shots.pdf.

Magalone, M., A. Ruelaz Maher, J. Hu, Z. Wang, R. Shanman, P. G. Shekelle, B. Roth, L. Hilton, M. J. Suttorp, B. A. Ewing, A. Motala, and T. Perry. "Off- Label Use of

Atypical Antipsychotics: An Update." *Comparative Effectiveness Review* 43 (September 2011). http://www.effectivehealthcare.ahrq.gov/ehc/products/150/778/CER43_Off-LabelAntipsychotics_20110928.pdf. Prepared for: Agency for Healthcare Research and Quality U.S. Department of Health and Human Service (AHRQ).

Mayden, Kelley D. "Peer Review: Publication's Gold Standard." *Journal of the Advanced Practitioner in Oncology* 3, no. 2 (2012): 117–22. Accessed March 19, 2015. doi:10.6004/jadpro.2012.3.2.8.

Miller, Neil Z., and Gary S. Goldman. "Infant Mortality Rates Regressed against Number of Vaccine Doses Routinely Given: Is There a Biochemical or Synergistic Toxicity?" *Human and Experimental Toxicology* 30, no. 9 (September 2011): 1420–428. Accessed September 14, 2013. doi:10.1177/0960327111407644.

Miller, Neil Z. *Vaccine Safety Manual for Concerned Families and Health Practitioners.* Santa Fe, NM: New Atlantean Press, 2010. 165–69.

Morgan Verkamp, LLC. "Statement of William W. Thompson, PhD., Regarding the 2004 Article Examining the Possibility of a Relationship between MMR Vaccine and Autism." News release, September 27, 2014. Morgan Verkamp. Accessed September 15, 2015. http://www.morganverkamp.com/august-27-2014-press-release-statement-of-william-w-thompson-ph-d.

National Institute of Infectious Disease. "Routine and Voluntary Vaccinations in Japan." Japan Healthcare Info. 2012. Accessed January 30, 2013. http://japanhealthinfo.com/child-health-and-childcare/vaccination/.

National Vaccine Information Center (NVIC). Accessed February 3, 2014. http://www.nvic.org/.

"National Vaccine Injury Compensation Program." Health Resources and Services Administration. Accessed October 8, 2015. http://www.hrsa.gov/vaccinecompensation/index.html.

"NDA 19-626/S-019." Robert Rappaport, MD to Pushpa Mehta, RAC. February 13, 2004. Rockville, MD: Food and Drug Administration. http://www.accessdata.fda.gov/drugsatfda_docs/appletter/2004/19626scs019ltr.pdf.

Offit, P. A., MD, and R. K. Jew, PharmD. "Addressing Parents' Concerns: Do Vaccines Contain Harmful Preservatives, Adjuvants, Additives, or Residuals?" *Pediatrics* 112, no. 6 (2003): 1394–397. doi:10.1542/peds.112.6.1394.

"Package Inserts and Manufacturers for Some US Licensed Vaccines and Immunoglobulins." Institute for Vaccine Safety at Johns Hopkins Bloomberg School of Public Health. Accessed February 3, 2014. http://www.vaccinesafety.edu/package_inserts.htm.

"Policies and Procedures for Handling Conflicts of Interest with FDA Advisory Committee Members, Consultants, and Experts." U.S. Food and Drug Administration. Accessed November 12, 2013. http://www.fda.gov/oc/advisory/conflictofinterest/policies.html.

"Poliomyelitis Prevention: Recommendations for Use of Inactivated Poliovirus Vaccine and Live Oral Poliovirus Vaccine." *Pediatrics* 99.2 (1997): 300–05. Print.

"Public Availability of Advisory Committee Members' Financial Interest Information and Waivers." U.S. Food and Drug Administration. Accessed March 18, 2015. http://www.fda.gov/RegulatoryInformation/Guidances/ucm391034.htm.

"Questions and Answers about Vaccine Ingredients." American Academy of Pediatrics. January 2013. https://www2.aap.org/immunization/families/faq/Vaccineingredients.pdf.

Redhead, K., G. J. Quinlan, R. G. Das, and J. M. C. Gutteridge. "Aluminium-Adjuvanted Vaccines Transiently Increase Aluminium Levels in Murine Brain Tissue." *Pharmacology & Toxicology* 70, no. 4 (1992): 278–80. doi:10.1111/j.1600-0773.1992.tb00471.x.

"Remove Vaccine Safety Oversight from DHHS." National Vaccine Information Center (NVIC). September 1, 2014. http://www.nvic.org/NVIC-Vaccine-News/September-2014/Remove-Vaccine-Safety-Oversight-From-DHHS.aspx.

"The Road to Safe and Effective Vaccines." PATH. April 2015. http://www.path.org/publications/files/VAC_clinical_trials_fs_2015.pdf.

Rosenbloom, Arlan L. "Hyperprolactinemia with Antipsychotic Drugs in Children and Adolescents." *International Journal of Pediatric Endocrinology* 2010 (2010): 1–6. doi:10.1155/2010/159402.

Sears, Robert W., MD, FAAP. *The Vaccine Book: Making the Right Decision for Your Child.* New York: Little, Brown, 2007.

The Side Effects of Common Psychiatric Drugs. PDF. Los Angeles: Citizens Commission on Human Rights, 2012.

Strebel, P. M., R. W. Sutter, S. L. Cochi, R. J. Biellik, E. W. Brink, O. M. Kew, M. A. Pallansch, W. A. Orenstein, and A. R. Hinman. "Epidemiology of Poliomyelitis in the United States One Decade after the Last Reported Case of Indigenous Wild Virus-Associated Disease." *Clinical Infectious Diseases* 14.2 (1992): 568–79. Print.

"Thimerosal (Mercury) Law." California Department of Public Health. Accessed January 28, 2014. http://www.cdph.ca.gov/programs/immunize/Pages/CaliforniaThimerosalLaw.aspx.

"Thimerosal in Vaccines." U.S. Food and Drug Administration. June 14, 2014. http://www.fda.gov/BiologicsBloodVaccines/SafetyAvailability/VaccineSafety/UCM096228#t1.

Tomljenovic, L., and C. A. Shaw. "Aluminum Vaccine Adjuvants: Are They Safe?" *Current Medicinal Chemistry CMC* 18, no. 17 (2011): 2630–637. doi:10.2174/092986711795933740.

Tomljenovic, L., and C. Shaw. "Mechanisms of Aluminum Adjuvant Toxicity and Autoimmunity in Pediatric Populations." *Lupus* 21, no. 2 (2012): 223–30. doi:10.1177/0961203311430221.

U.S. Congress. House. Government Reform. *FACA: Conflicts of Interest and Vaccine Development—Preserving the Integrity of the Process.* 106 Cong., 2d sess. H. Rept. Serial No. 106-239. June 15, 2000. http://www.gpo.gov/fdsys/pkg/CHRG-106hhrg73042/html/CHRG-106hhrg73042.htm.

U.S. Congress. House. Government Reform. *Mercury in Medicine—Taking Unnecessary Risks.* By Dan Burton. 106 Cong. H. Rept. 76. Vol. 149. Government Printing Office, 2003. http://www.gpo.gov/.

"U.S. Meat Production." Physicians for Social Responsibility. Accessed May 21, 2013. http://www.psr.org/chapters/oregon/safe-food/industrial-meat-system.html.

United States. Centers for Disease Control and Prevention. Management Analysis and Services. *Federal Advisory Committee Management Handbook.* 2008. Accessed February 27, 2015. http://www.cdc.gov/maso/facm/pdfs/Committeehandbook.pdf.

United States. Department of Health and Human Services. Health Resources and Services Administration. *HRSA.gov.* May 4, 2015. Accessed May 15, 2015 and December 13, 2016. http://www.hrsa.gov/vaccinecompensation/statisticsreport.pdf.

United States. Department of Health and Human Services. Office of Inspector General. *CDC's Ethics Program for Special Government Employees on Federal Advisory Committees.* Accessed February 25, 2015. http://oig.hhs.gov/oei/reports/oei-04-07-00260.pdf.

United States. Department of Health and Human Services. U.S. Food and Drug Administration. *Agency Information Collection Activities; Submission for OMB Review; Comment Request; Aluminum in Large and Small Volume Parenterals Used in Total Parenteral Nutrition.* March 10, 2003. http://www.fda.gov/ohrms/dockets/98fr/oc0367.pdf.

"Update on Recommendations for the Use of Rotavirus Vaccines." Archived Content. U.S. Food and Drug Administration. May 14, 2010. http://www.fda.gov/BiologicsBloodVaccines/Vaccines/ApprovedProducts/ucm212140.htm.

"Vaccine Adverse Event Reporting System (VAERS)." Centers for Disease Control and Prevention. July 24, 2013. Accessed April 15, 2014. http://www.cdc.gov/vaccinesafety/Activities/vaers.html.

"Vaccine Exemptions." Institute for Vaccine Safety. Accessed March 23, 2015. http://www.vaccinesafety.edu/cc-exem.htm.

Vaccine Information Statement Polio-OPV Supplement. Washington D.C.: U.S. Department of Health and Human Services Centers for Disease Control and Prevention National Immunization Program, 2000. Print.

"Vaccine Safety Questions and Answers." U.S. Food and Drug Administration. Accessed February 25, 2015. http://www.fda.gov/BiologicsBloodVaccines/SafetyAvailability/VaccineSafety/ucm133806.htm.

"Vaccines Licensed for Immunization and Distribution in the U.S. with Supporting Documents." U.S. Food and Drug Administration. Accessed March 3, 2015. http://www.fda.gov/BiologicsBloodVaccines/Vaccines/ApprovedProducts/ucm093830.htm.

"Vaccines." U.S. Food and Drug Administration. Accessed May 30, 2014. http://www.fda.gov/BiologicsBloodVaccines/Vaccines/default.htm.

"VIS Frequently Asked Questions." Centers for Disease Control and Prevention. April 30, 2015. Accessed November 14, 2014. http://www.cdc.gov/vaccines/hcp/vis/about/vis-faqs.html.

"What Are 'Biologics' Questions and Answers." U.S. Food and Drug Administration. Accessed September 19, 2014. http://www.fda.gov/AboutFDA/CentersOffices/OfficeofMedicalProductsandTobacco/CBER/ucm133077.htm.

Chapter 7

"A Toxic Flood." Food & Water Watch. May 16, 2013. Accessed August 2, 2013. http://www.foodandwaterwatch.org/reports/a-toxic-flood/.

"About Air Toxics." U.S. Environmental Protection Agency. Accessed September 11, 2013. http://www.epa.gov/air/toxicair/newtoxics.html.

"About Sewage Sludge." Center for Food Safety. Accessed October 1, 2013. http://www.centerforfoodsafety.org/issues/1050/sewage-sludge/about-sewage-sludge.

Alberta, Lauren, Susan Sweeney, MD, and Karen Wiss, MD. "Diaper Dye Dermatitis." *Pediatrics* 116, no. 3 (September 01, 2005): E450–452. doi:10.1542/peds.2004-2066.

Anderson, Rosalind C., and Julius H. Anderson. "Acute Respiratory Effects of Diaper Emissions." *Archives of Environmental Health: An International* Journal 54, no. 5 (September/October 1999): 353–58. doi:10.1080/00039899909602500.

Arkin, Lisa, Executive Director, Beyond Toxics. "West Eugene Air Pollution." E-mail message to author, Joanne Stanton. October 18, 2013.http://www.easybib.com/cite/view

Avril, Tom, and Jennifer Moroz. "Toms River Families Settle Cancer Claims A Mediated Deal Covers 69 Families That Blamed Companies for Their Children's Illnesses. Suits Are Pending in Separate Cases." *Philadelphia Inquirer*, December 14, 2001. http://articles.philly.com/2001-12-14/news/25307892_1_cancer-claims-families-separate-cases.

Back-to-School Guide to PVC-Free School Supplies. The Center for Health, Environment & Justice Guide. August 2013. Accessed October 23, 2013. http://www.chej.org/publications/PVCGuide/PVCfree.pdf.

"Basics of Green Chemistry." U.S. Environmental Protection Agency. Accessed October 23, 2013. http://www2.epa.gov/green-chemistry/basics-green-chemistry#definition.

"Body Burden: The Pollution in Newborns." Environmental Working Group. July 2005. Accessed October 20, 2013. http://www.ewg.org/research/body-burden-pollution-newborns.

"Body Burden: The Pollution in People." Environmental Working Group. Accessed October 24, 2013. http://www.ewg.org/sites/bodyburden1/findings.php.

"Camp Lejeune Marine Corps Base Jacksonville, NC." Military Base Contamination Bell Legal Group. Accessed October 01, 2015. http://www.militarycontamination.com/JacksonvilleNC.php.

Center for Food Safety. "Chemical Corporations Undermine the Will of the People of Hawaii County." News release, November 26, 2014. http://www.centerforfoodsafety.org/press-releases/3628/chemical-corporations-undermine-the-will-of-the-people-of-hawaii-county.

CFC SB 772 Fact Sheet: Toxic Flame Retardants and Fire Safety Alternatives." Consumer Federation of California. August 12, 2007. http://consumercal.org/cfc-sb-772-fact-sheet-toxic-flame-retardants-and-fire-safety-alternatives/.

Christopher S. Crockett, PhD, PE, Deputy Water Commissioner. "Philadelphia Water Authority—Comments on the Application for Phase I Criteria Siting Permit by Elcon Recycling Services, LLC." Philadelphia Water Authority. November 14, 2015. Accessed November 20, 2015. http://www.phila.gov/water/PDF/PhiladelphiaWater_Elcon.ph1Permit_Comments.pdf.

"The Clean Air Act." Union of Concerned Scientists. February 1, 2012. http://www.ucsusa.org/global_warming/solutions/big_picture_solutions/the-clean-air-act.html.

"Clean Water Action Alert: Help Protect Water from Toxic Power Plant Pollution." Clean Water Action. Spring 2015. Accessed June 27, 2015. www.cleanwateraction.org.

"Congress Must Act to Remove Toxic Substances from Products Our Families Use Everyday: Flame Retardants TDCP and TCEP." National Resources Defense Council. July 2010. Accessed August 30, 2013. http://www.nrdc.org/health/flameretardants-fs.asp.

"Contaminants of Concern at Camp Lejeune Military Res. (USNAVY) EPA." United States Environmental Protection Agency. November 10, 2015. Accessed January/February, 2015. http://cumulis.epa.gov/supercpad/SiteProfiles/index.cfm?fuseaction=second.Contams&id=0403185.

"Current Drinking Water Regulations." U.S. Environmental Protection Agency. March 6, 2012. Accessed September 23, 2013. http://water.epa.gov/lawsregs/rulesregs/sdwa/currentregulations.cfm.

Cuthert, Donna, Vice President, The Alliance For a Clean Environment. "Excelon Release Reports from Limerick Nuclear Power Plant." E-mail message to author, Joanne Stanton. October 22, 2013.

"Disease Clusters Spotlight the Need to Protect People from Toxic Chemicals." National Resources Defense Council. Accessed May 10, 2011. http://www.nrdc.org/health/diseaseclusters.

"Environmental Chemicals Harm Reproductive Health." American Congress of Obstetricians and Gynecologists. September 23, 2013. Accessed October 25, 2013. http://www.acog.org/About_ACOG/News_Room/News_Releases/2013/Environmental_Chemicals_Harm_Reproductive_Health.

"Environmental Justice Case Study: Shintech PVC Plant in Convent, Louisiana." University of Michigan. Accessed October 20, 201. http://www.umich.edu/~snre492/shin.html.

"Environmentally Benign Products: A Green Chemistry Mentor Speaks." Social Climate Group. July 27, 2011. Accessed October 23, 2013. http://socialclimate.wordpress.com/2011/07/27/environmentally-benign-products-a-green-chemistry-mentor-speaks/.

"EPA Emerging Contaminants Fact Sheet PFOA and PFOS." U.S. Environmental Protection Agency. March 2013. Accessed September 05, 2015. http://www2.epa.gov/sites/production/files/documents/ec_technical_fs_pfos_pfoa_march_2013.pdf.

"EPA Superfund Program: Camp Lejeune Military Res. (USNAVY), Onslow County, NC." United States Environmental Protection Agency. Accessed September 15, 2015. http://cumulis.epa.gov/supercpad/cursites/csitinfo.cfm?id=0403185.

"EPA To Develop Regulation for Perchlorate." U.S. Environmental Protection Agency. February 2, 2011. Accessed September 24, 2013. http://yosemite.epa.gov/opa/admpress.nsf/1e5ab1124055f3b28525781f0042ed40/6348845793f4c c5d8525782b004d81ae%21OpenDocument.

"EWG's Guide to Safe Drinking Water." Environmental Working Group. Accessed September 6, 2013. http://www.ewg.org/research/ewgs-guide-safe-drinking-water.

Fagan, John, Michael Antonio, and Claire Robinson. *GMO Myths and Truths. An Evidence-based Examination of GMO Claims (Second Edition)* pg. 221. Report. London: Earth Open Source, 2012. Accessed May 20, 2015. http://earthopensource.org/wp-content/uploads/2014/11/GMO-Myths-and-Truths-edition2.pdf.

Fiedler, Heidelore. *Dioxin and Furan Inventories National and Regional Emissions of PCDD/PCDF.* May 1999. United Nations Environment Programme (UNEP) Chemicals, Geneva, Switzerland. Available online at: http://www.unep.org/chemicalsandwaste/portals/9/POPs/Toolkit-Inventories/difurpt.pdf

"Gathering Dust: Many Toxic Flame Retardants Linger in Homes, Sometimes at Levels Above Health Guidelines." Silent Spring Institute. Accessed September 16, 2013. http://www.silentspring.org/our-research/research-updates/gathering-dust-many-toxic-flame-retardants-linger-homes-sometimes-leve.

"Ground Water." U.S. Environmental Protection Agency. March 6, 2012. Accessed September 10, 2013. http://water.epa.gov/type/groundwater/index.cfm.

Guzman, Alison, and Lisa Arkin. *Environmental Justice in West Eugene: Families, Health, and Air Pollution.* Grant Report for the US EPA Environmental Justice Small Grant Program. Eugene, OR: Beyond Toxics, 2011-2012.

"HAZARD ALERT—Worker Exposure to Silica during Hydraulic Fracturing." Occupational & Safety and Health Administration. June 2012. https://www.osha.gov/dts/hazardalerts/hydraulic_frac_hazard_alert.html.

"Hidden Radioactive Releases from Nuclear Power Plants in the United States." Nuclear Information and Resource Service. November 2005. Accessed October 10, 2013. http://www.nirs.org/factsheets/drey_usa_pamphlet.pdf.

Horwitt, Dusty. "Methane Hunt Shines Light on Natural Gas." *Environmental Working Group's EnviroBlog,* April 12, 2013. Accessed August 2, 2013. http://www.ewg.org/enviroblog/2013/04/methane-hunt-shines-light-natural-gas.

"How to Read Your Water Quality Report." Food & Water Watch. Accessed September 12, 2013. http://www.foodandwaterwatch.org/water/triclosan/water-quality-report/.

Imus, Deirdre. *Growing up Green: Baby and Childcare.* Vol. 2. New York, NY: Simon & Schuster, 2008. 11.

"Letter Health Consultation: Water Analysis of Private Wells Located within Proximity of Salford Quarry Superfund Site." Pauline Risser-Clemens, Health Assessor, Health Assessment Program, Division of Environmental Health Epidemiology to Sharon Fang, Remedial Project Manager, US EPA Region 3. November 01, 2012. Prepared by *Pennsylvania Department of Health Division of Environmental Health Epidemiology Under Cooperative Agreement with the U.S. Department of Health and Human Services Agency for*

Toxic Substances and Disease Registry. Accessed October 01, 2015. http://www.atsdr.cdc.gov/HAC/pha/SalfordQuarry/SalfordQuarryLHCfinalrelease10312012.pdf.

"Limerick Nuclear Power Plant License Renewal Is NOT Good For Your Health, Safety, or Environment." The Alliance for a Clean Environment. Accessed May 1, 2013. http://www.acereport.org/.

Lochbaum, David. *Regulatory Roulette: The NRC's Inconsistent Oversight of Radioactive Releases from Nuclear Power Plants.* Report. Union of Concerned Scientists. September 2010. Accessed 18 December 2016. http://www.ucsusa.org/sites/default/files/legacy/assets/documents/nuclear_power/nuclear-power-radioactive-releases.pdf

Lowman, Amy, Mary Anne McDonald, Steve Wing, and Naeema Muhammad. "Land Application of Treated Sewage Sludge: Community Health and Environmental Justice." *Environmental Health Perspectives* 121, no. 5 (2013): 537–42. doi:10.1289/ehp.1205470.

Mangano, Joseph J. *Health Hazards to Fetuses, Infants, and Young Children in Heavily-fracked Areas of Pennsylvania.* Report. New York: Radiation and Public Health Project, 2015.

Mangano, Joseph J., Jay M. Gould, Ernest J. Sternglass, Janette D. Sherman, and William Mcdonnell. "An Unexpected Rise in Strontium-90 in U.S. Deciduous Teeth in the 1990s." *Science of The Total Environment* 317, no. 1-3 (2003): 37–51. doi:10.1016/S0048-9697(03)00439-X.

Mott, Lawrie, David Fore, Jennifer Curtis, and Gina Solomon. "Our Children At Risk: The Five Worst Environmental Threats to Their Health." National Resources Defense Council. November 1997. http://www.nrdc.org/health/kids/ocar/ocarinx.asp.

"Myths & Realities of GE Crops." Center for Food Safety. Accessed February 18, 2015. http://www.centerforfoodsafety.org/issues/311/ge-foods/myths-and-realities-of-ge-crops.

"Naval Air Development Center: 24 Bases with Reported TCE Water Contamination." Military Base Contamination Bell Legal Group. Accessed November 12, 2015. http://www.militarycontamination.com/WarminsterTownshipPA.php.

Nazaryan, Alexander. "Camp Lejeune and the U.S. Military's Polluted Legacy." *Newsweek*, July 25, 2014. Accessed September 15, 2015. http://www.newsweek.com/2014/07/25/us-military-supposed-protect-countrys-citizens-and-soldiers-not-poison-them-259103.html.

Neuhauser, Alan. "Behind New York's Fracking Ban." *U.S. News and World Report.* December 19, 2014. Accessed February 02, 2015. http://www.usnews.com/news/articles/2014/12/19/behind-new-yorks-fracking-ban.

"New York Residents Present Gov. Cuomo with Over 200,000 Petitions Calling for a Ban on Fracking." New Yorkers against Fracking. Accessed October 10, 2013. http://nyagainstfracking.org/new-york-residents-present-gov-cuomo-with-over-200000-petitions-calling-for-a-ban-on-fracking/.

Nuclear Power and Children. A Fact Sheet from Beyondnuclear.org. June 2013. Accessed August 12, 2013. http://www.beyondnuclear.org/storage/radiation-and-health/radchild.pdf.

Ostroff. "Fracking: Dangerous to the Environment." Fracident Injury Law. Accessed September 22, 2013. http://frackinginjurylaw.com/fracking-dangers/?gclid=CLHP9_Wu4rkCFVGe4Aod_GIAUw.

"Persistent, Bioaccumulative, and Toxic Chemicals (PBTs)." Safer Chemicals, Healthy Families. Accessed October 1, 2013. http://saferchemicals.org/get-the-facts/chemicals-of-concern/persistent-bioaccumulative-and-toxic-chemicals-pbts/.

Pesticide Tolerances: Glyphosate. [Public Docket ID: EPA-HQ-OPP-2012-0132], U.S. Environmental Protection Agency (May 1, 2013). Accessed at: http://www.regulations.gov/#%21documentDetail;D=EPA-HQ-OPP-2012-0132-0009

Peterson, Iver. "Study Ties Childhood Cancer In Toms River to Pollution." *New York Times*, December 18, 2001. Accessed September 01, 2015. http://www.nytimes.com/2001/12/18/nyregion/study-ties-childhood-cancer-in-toms-river-to-pollution.html.

"Protecting Children and Communities from Disease Clusters." National Disease Clusters Alliance. August 2, 2012. Accessed October 28, 2013.

"PVC The Poison Plastic." Center for Health Environment Justice. Accessed October 23, 2013. http://chej.org/campaigns/pvc/.

Radiation and Public Health Project. "Pennsylvania Study Links Fracking to Health Hazards in Fetuses, Infants, and Young Children." News release, July 26, 2015. EIN Presswire. http://www.einpresswire.com/article/277887528/pennsylvania-study-links-fracking-to-health-hazards-in-fetuses-infants-and-young-children.

"Radionuclides in Drinking Water: Reverse Osmosis." U.S. Environmental Protection Agency. Accessed May 05, 2015. http://cfpub.epa.gov/safewater/radionuclides/radionuclides.cfm?action=Rad_Reverse+Osmosis.

Samsel, Anthony, and Stephanie Seneff. "Glyphosate's Suppression of Cytochrome P450 Enzymes and Amino Acid Biosynthesis by the Gut Microbiome: Pathways to Modern Diseases." *Entropy* 15, no. 4 (2013): 1416–463. doi:10.3390/e15041416.

Saunders, Norman R., Shane A. Liddelow, and Katarzyna M. Dziegielewska. "Barrier Mechanisms in the Developing Brain." *Frontiers in Pharmacology* 3 (2012). Accessed September 13, 20132. doi:10.3389/fphar.2012.00046.

Schramm, Josh. "ToxicNursery-01.jpg." Digital image. Washington Toxics Coalition. Accessed December 12, 2013. www.watoxics.org.

"Science, Democracy, and Fracking: A Guide for Community Residents and Policy Makers Facing Decisions over Hydraulic Fracturing." Union of Concerned Scientists. September 10, 2013. Accessed September 20, 2013. http://www.ucsusa.org/center-for-science-and-democracy/events/fracking-forum-toolkit.html.

Sesana, Laura. "EPA Raises Levels of Glyphosate Residue Allowed in Food." *Washington Times Communities*, July 5, 2013. Accessed July 22, 2013. http://communities.washingtontimes.com/neighborhood/world-our-backyard/2013/jul/5/epa-raises-levels-glyphosate-residue-allowed-your-/.

"Sixty-eight Public Interest Groups Applaud Senator Boxer's Investigation and Hearings on Toxics in Drinking Water and Sewage Sludge Poisoning Our Food." Center for Food Safety. April 15, 2008. Accessed October 12, 1012. http://www.centerforfoodsafety.org/press-releases/841/sixty-eight-public-interest-groups-applaud-senator-boxers-investigation-and-hearings-on-toxics-in-drinking-water-and-sewage-sludge-poisoning-our-food. http://www.easybib.com/cite/view

Skelton, Renee, and Vernice Miller. "The Environmental Justice Movement." National Resources Defense Council. October 12, 2006. Accessed October 12, 2013. http://www.nrdc.org/ej/history/hej.asp.

Snyder, Caroline, PhD. "The Dirty Work of Promoting 'Recycling' of America's Sewage Sludge." *International Journal of Occupational Medicine and Environmental Health*. 11, no. 4 (October 2005): 415–27. http://www.sludgefacts.org/IJOEH_1104_Snyder.pdf.

The Story of Stuff. By Annie Leonard and Jonah Sachs. Directed by Louis Fox. Performed by Annie Leonard. Free Range Studios. December 2007. Accessed November 01, 2013. http://storyofstuff.org/movies/story-of-stuff/.

Tatu, Christina. "Communities Can Do Little to Keep PennEast Pipeline out." *The Morning Call* (Allentown: Community News Northampton), June 15, 2015.

Teller, Suzanne. "The Clean Water Act: 40 Years of Progress in Peril." *Outdoor America*, 2012. Accessed September 12, 2013. http://www.iwla.org/index.php?ht=action/ GetDocumentAction/i/50660.

United States. Agency for Toxic Substances and Disease Registry. Department of Health and Human Services. Federal Facilities Assessment Branch. Division of Health Assessment and Consultation. *Willow Grove Naval Air Station/Air Reserve Station Public Health Assessment.* May 2002. Accessed September 01, 2015. http://www.atsdr.cdc.gov/HAC/pha/ WillowGrove051602-PA/WillowGrove051602-PA.pdf.

United States. Agency for Toxic Substances and Disease Registry. U.S. Department of Health and Human Services. Federal Facilities Assessment Branch. Division of Health Assessment and Consultation. *Naval Air Warfare Center Public Health Assessment.* October 25, 2002. Accessed September 01, 2015. http://www.atsdr.cdc.gov/hac/pha/pha. asp?docid=351&pg=0.

United States. Department of Health and Human Services. National Cancer Institute. *Reducing Environmental Cancer Risk, What We Can Do Now—2008–2009 Annual Report President's Cancer Panel.* By Suzanne H. Reuben. April 2010. http://deainfo.nci.nih.gov/advisory/pcp/ annualReports/pcp08-09rpt/PCP_Report_08-09_508.pdf.

United States. Environmental Protection Agency and Centers for Disease Control Agency for Toxic Substance. National Service Center for Environmental Publications. *Trichloroethylene (TCE) TEACH Chemical Summary.* 2007. Accessed August 05, 2015. http://nepis.epa.gov/ Exe/ZyPURL.cgi?Dockey=P100BNS7.txt.

United States Environmental Protection Agency. "Emerging Contaminants Fact Sheet— PFOS and PFOA." *Emerging Contaminants—Perfluorooctane Sulfonate (PFOS) and Perfluorooctanoic Acid (PFOA),* March 2014. http://www2.epa.gov/sites/production/ files/2014-04/documents/factsheet_contaminant_pfos_pfoa_march2014.pdf.

United States Environmental Protection Agency. Region 3. "Salford Quarry Site Added to Superfund List." News release, September 23, 2009. EPA. Accessed August 05, 2015. http://yosemite.epa.gov/opa/admpress.nsf.

"Video: 10 Americans." Environmental Working Group. July 23, 2012. Accessed October 20, 2013. http://www.ewg.org/news/videos/10-americans.

Walker, Bill. "RE: Mother and Author seeking permission and advice." E-mail message to author, Joanne Stanton. October 23, 2013.

"Water." Pollution Facts, Effects of Pollution, Clean Act. Accessed August 25, 2013. http://www. nrdc.org/water/.

"What Is Environmental Medicine?" American Academy of Environmental Medicine. Accessed August 11, 2013. http://www.aaemonline.org/introduction.html.

"What Is Green Power?" U.S Department of Energy. February 11, 2013. Accessed September 2, 2013. http://apps3.eere.energy.gov/greenpower/buying.

"What's at Risk from Industry's Full-Scale Assault on the EPA and the Clean Air Act?" National Resources Defense Council. December 2, 2010. Accessed October 14, 2013. http://www. nrdc.org/air/cleanairact/default.asp.

White, Heather. "Chemical Industry to Pregnant Women: Don't Worry Your Pretty Little Heads." *Environmental Working Group's EnviroBlog,* September 24, 2013. Accessed September 28, 2013. http://www.ewg.org/enviroblog/2013/09/chemical-industry-pregnant-women-don-t-worry-your-pretty-little-heads.

World Health Organization. The International Agency for Research on Cancer. "IARC Monographs Volume 112: Evaluation of Five Organophosphate Insecticides and Herbicides." News release, March 20, 2015. Accessed May 01, 2015. http://www.iarc.fr/en/ media-centre/iarcnews/pdf/MonographVolume112.pdf.

Zerbo, Advocacy Coordinator, Russell. "Clean Air Council of Philadelphia Public Comment on the Application for Phase I Criteria Siting Permit by Elcon Recycling Services, LLC." Delaware River Keeper. October 30, 2015. Accessed November 20, 2015. http://www.delawareriverkeeper.org/Documents/Clean%20Air%20Council%20PADEP%20Comment%209.30.2015.pdf.

Chapter 9

Burton's Legal Thesaurus, 4E. S.v. "loophole." Retrieved April 2, 2015, from http://legal-dictionary.thefreedictionary.com/loophole.

Collins, Ronald K . L., and Paul McMasters. "Veggie-Libel Law Still Poses a Threat." Center for Science in the Public Interest. FoodSpeak Free Speech Project: Collins & McMasters Legal Times Op Ed. Accessed May 20, 2015. http://www.cspinet.org/foodspeak/oped/candm.htm.

"Existing Food-Disparagement Laws by State." Center for Science in the Public Interest. FoodSpeak Free Speech Project. Accessed May 05, 2014. http://cspinet.org/foodspeak/laws/existlaw.htm.

"Government-Industry Revolving Door." SourceWatch. Accessed May 20, 2015. http://www.sourcewatch.org/index.php?title=Government-industry_revolving_door.

Lindbloom, Isaac, and Kelly Terranova. Summary Citizens United v. Federal Election Commission (Docket No. 08-205). Cornell University School of Law School. Legal Information Institute Supreme Court Bulletin. Edited by Hana Bae. Accessed May 20, 2015. https://www.law.cornell.edu/supct/cert/08-205.

"Lobbying." Encyclopedia Britannica. Accessed May 20, 2015. http://www.britannica.com/EBchecked/topic/345407/lobbying.

"Revolving Door." Opensecrets. Center for Responsive Politics. Accessed May 04, 2014. http://www.opensecrets.org/revolving.

Story of Citizens United v. FEC—The Story of Stuff Project. By Annie Leonard, Jonah Sachs, and Lois Fox. Directed by Lois Fox. Produced by Free Range Studios. Performed by Annie Leonard. The Story of Stuff Project. June 01, 2012. http://storyofstuff.org/movies/story-of-citizens-united-v-fec/.

Tsukayama, Hayley. "FCC Commissioner Meredith Baker to Join Comcast-NBC." *Washington Post.* May 13, 2011. Accessed May 04, 2014. http://www.washingtonpost.com/blogs/post-tech/post/fcc-commissioner-meredith-baker-to-join-comcast-nbc/2011/05/11/AFYfl1rG_blog.html.

West's Encyclopedia of American Law, edition 2. S.v. "rider." Retrieved April 2, 2015, from http://legal-dictionary.thefreedictionary.com/rider.

"What Is Lobbying?" Association of Government Relations Professionals. June 27, 2013. Accessed April 02, 2015. http://grprofessionals.org/about-lobbying/what-is-lobbying.

RESOURCE GUIDE

Like Abraham Lincoln, I am a firm believer in the people. If given the truth, they can be depended upon to meet any national crisis. The great point is to bring them the real facts.
—General Douglas MacArthur

We put this Resource Guide together so that you have a starting point for additional information on many of the book's topics. We hope it empowers you to connect with the numerous organizations and government agencies listed and take advantage of the many valuable online tools they offer.

Also, we'll be continually updating the Resource Guide as we get new information, so go to www.behindcloseddoorsthebook.com to download a free electronic copy of the most up-to-date version and sign up to be notified whenever a new version is released.

Resources for Chapters 1 to 4

Background Information on Children's Health Statistics
As mentioned in Chapter 3, "The Changing State of Children's Health," finding statistics on children's health conditions in the United States is not as simple as you would think. Understandably, certain areas of our nation's health are tracked more closely than others. For instance, reportable diseases (such as meningitis) and foodborne illnesses (such as *E. coli*) are required by law to be reported and tracked at the state level, and then at the national level once a case is confirmed. This is because they are communicable illnesses that can spread quickly across various communities. However, you may be very surprised to learn that most health conditions, such as diabetes, asthma, autism, depression, etc., are not required to be reported to anyone, at any level. Many barriers exist to collecting this vital information. As a result, there is no national registry, or single center of data collection, that houses the actual "real" number of children afflicted with these types of health conditions during a given year. With no true raw data available for the book (e.g., 1 million cases of asthma in children age 18 and under in 1980), we needed to find the most reliable methods to obtain the statistical estimates we needed.

Researchers use a variety of ways to collect data (such as surveys or scientific studies) on a specific population (such as children with asthma) from various people or places (such as parents, doctors, or hospitals) to make estimates about the number of new cases (known as incidence) or new and existing cases (known as prevalence) in a particular location (United States) at a given point in time (1980 or 2010). Surveys and scientific research studies are two of the most common methods used by researchers to collect this type of health information at a local, state, or national level.

Various organizations and U.S. government agencies, such as the Centers for Disease Control and Prevention (CDC) and the National Institutes of Health (NIH), currently follow certain selected children's health statistics using a variety of national health surveys. These surveys collect health information from a small sample of people as a starting point to provide statistical estimates on various aspects of these childhood health conditions in the United States. Asthma is one example of a childhood health condition being tracked through national surveys. Asthma is monitored because it affects a large number of children and is known to have various environmental triggers that may be controllable.

In recent years the CDC has also started to track childhood diabetes and autism spectrum disorder at selected sites across the country due to growing concern of increasing incidence rates. But outside of these national surveys and surveillance studies we rely heavily on experts in various fields of health and science to conduct and publish studies in peer-reviewed medical journals that provide us with additional opportunities to obtain reliable estimates and deeper insight into children's health conditions.

Challenges to the Statistics We Needed

We always attempted to find studies and surveys that provided the highest data reliability for this book. Most often, due to limited data on childhood health conditions, we had to use what researchers in various fields of study consider the best existing data. An example of this would be childhood diabetes data from registries in Philadelphia and Wisconsin that has provided medical researchers and public health officials with the best existing data from the past twenty years to make estimates on the increase in childhood diabetes in the United States. But remember, registries are few and far between for most childhood conditions. Many other childhood disorders that have recently skyrocketed, such as bipolar disorder, often do not receive the same research attention as diabetes because the condition affects fewer children. As a result, a random study here or there is the only window we have into the incidence or prevalence at a certain point in time. Often the data we had to compare was not the ideal comparison but rather the only comparison we could find to try to make general estimates on changes in the health of our children over time.

How Important Is Statistical Data from Research?

When barriers exist to tracking valuable health information it often impedes efforts to identify trends in health statistics for implementing intervention programs. Those working in the field of medical research have been pleading for a more coordinated effort in the area of health data collection for quite some time. Reliable statistical data from research provides valuable health information. This information is then used to help public health officials, scientists, and medical personnel track, study, and evaluate the health of children in the United States.

The statistical data obtained serves as evidence that a problem exists and allows researchers to build upon basic research with new, larger studies to find solutions to the problems. An example of problems discovered through research would be finding a sudden increase in the number of children diagnosed with a particular condition (autism) or that a major health disparity exists within the condition, such as a disparity in gender (autism affects more boys than girls), or race (autism affects mostly whites), or place of residence (autism affects a larger percentage of children living in California than any other state). It is only when awareness of a particular health problem has been established that funding for education, support programs, and additional research may be initiated.

Where Does Research Funding Come From?

The two main sources of funding for health-related research studies are large corporations and the government. Large corporations usually fund research through their research and development departments, while the government usually carries funding out through universities and special government agencies. Fewer research dollars come from sources such as nonprofit organizations and private donations. Funding for research is a highly competitive process. Research projects are evaluated by those sponsoring the study, and often only a select few studies ever receive funding. Generally speaking, children's health issues don't always get the same research attention as adult health issues because funding tends to be based on numbers. Children in the United States are a smaller population than adults in the United States and traditionally have fewer health problems than adults. Therefore, spending money and resources to help fewer people would not make the *economic sense* of spending the same money to help more people.

Many of the studies conducted in smaller health populations, such as children with food allergies, tend to be funded by corporations or special interest groups. These special interest groups have a vested interest in some aspect of the research. The most obvious business interest is the potential to make a profit. Therefore, very costly research into childhood food allergies that could potentially result in anaphylaxic shock takes place because a lifesaving product, such as EpiPen, is in research and development. If these same corporations do not feel their costly research will result in large enough profits (translation: not enough children are affected), valuable research may never be conducted. This is why we need more research dollars allocated to children's health . . . so that important research (such as SEARCH for diabetes) can be conducted for additional health conditions affecting our children.

Seek and You Shall Find

Ironically, and true to the message within this book about the power of money, when we could not obtain relevant statistical information in the published medical journals we decided to search financial data to see if that avenue held statistics on any childhood illnesses. B-I-N-G-O! When we started looking at data provided by the U.S. Medical Expenditure Panel Survey (who tracks where our health spending dollars go) and the U.S. Department of Education (who needs to track every dollar spent on special education services). Additional health data surfaced by doing nothing more than following the money trail.

President's Cancer Panel Recommendations to Reduce Cancer Risks

According to the President's Cancer Panel, there are many things we can do to protect our families from cancer. Below are some of the 2010 report recommendations to reduce cancer risks for children and families, reprinted with their permission:

- Use filtered tap water or filtered well water instead of commercially bottled water to reduce exposure to numerous known or suspected carcinogens and endocrine-disrupting chemicals (unless the home water source is known to be contaminated).
- Storing and carrying water in stainless steel, glass, or BPA- and phthalate-free containers will reduce exposure from endocrine-disrupting and other chemicals that can leach into water from plastic.
- Family exposure to occupational chemicals can be reduced by removing shoes before entering the home and washing work clothes separately from the rest of the family laundry.

- Microwaving food in ceramic or glass instead of plastic containers will reduce exposure to endocrine-disrupting chemicals that may leach into food when containers are heated.
- Exposure to pesticides can be decreased by choosing, to the extent possible, food grown without pesticides or chemical fertilizers and washing conventionally grown produce to remove residues.
- Similarly, exposure to antibiotics, growth hormones, and toxic runoff from livestock feedlots can be minimized by eating free-range meat raised without these medications.
- Avoiding or minimizing consumption of processed, charred, and well-done meats will reduce exposure to carcinogenic agents (amines and polyaromatic hydrocarbons).
- Choose products made with nontoxic substances or environmentally friendly chemicals. Consult information sources such as the Household Products Database to help make informed decisions about products purchased and used.
- Reducing or ceasing the use of landscaping pesticides and fertilizers will help keep these chemicals from contaminating drinking-water supplies.
- Reduce or eliminate exposure to secondhand tobacco smoke in your home and auto and in public places.
- Children can reduce their radiation exposure to electromagnetic energy by wearing a headset when using a cell phone, texting instead of calling, and keeping calls brief.
- To reduce exposures to radiation from medical imaging, discuss with your healthcare provider the need for medical tests or procedures that involve radiation exposure. Key considerations include the patient history of radiation exposure, the expected benefits of the test, and alternative ways of obtaining the same information. To limit cumulative exposure, keep records of all imaging or nuclear medicine tests received and, if known, the estimated exposure dose for each test.
- Periodically check home radon levels.
- Avoid exposure to ultraviolet light by wearing protective clothing and sunscreens when outdoor and avoid exposure when the sunlight is most intense.

TSCA Reform

An easy-to-read abbreviated guide to TSCA Reform (the Frank R. Lautenberg Chemical Safety for the 21st Century Act) can be found on the website of Safer Chemicals, Healthy Families at saferchemicals.org/get-the-facts. More detailed information on Safer Chemicals, Healthy Families can be found in the resources for Chapters 7 and 8.

Resources for Chapter 5: Food

Processed Food

Center for Science in the Public Interest (CSPI)

The CSPI website (www.cspinet.org) provides helpful information on eating healthy. Their resource library includes additional reading on food dyes and the relationship between diet and behavior. It also includes health reports and even a food coloring database. Here you can check out "A Parent's Guide to Diet, ADHD and Behaviors." The CSPI is one of the nation's top consumer advocates "fighting for government policies and corporate practices that promote healthy diets, prevent deceptive marketing practices, and ensure that science is used to promote the public's welfare." Just a few of CSPI's accomplishments include leading the efforts to win passage of laws that require nutrition facts on packaged foods (and, later, to include trans-fat on those labels), defining the term "organic" for foods, and placing warning notices on alcoholic beverages.

Food Additives and GRAS Label

The FDA is responsible for determining the safety of food additives. A label commonly used for food additives is GRAS (generally regarded as safe), which indicates a widely used food additive believed to be safe enough to be exempt from further testing. Standards for GRAS have been tightened over the past few decades, but many loopholes still exist.

The infographic shown below, courtesy of the Center for Science in the Public Interest (CSPI), shows how companies get a food additive approved for their food item. Visit CSPI to get involved in efforts to change this system.

Special Diets for Special Kids (Volumes 1 and 2)

This comprehensive and easy-to-read book by Dr. Lisa Lewis is a great resource and a must-have if you have a child with medical conditions. Her son's diagnosis of autism and his success with dietary interventions led her to write this award-winning book series. It includes many recipes as well as simplified scientific research supporting the connections between nutrition and a variety of childhood diseases and disorders. Specific nutritional advice is provided for many health conditions, and many hopeful stories are shared of how simply changing your diet can improve (and sometimes even cure) common health problems in children. Below is a brief list from Dr. Lisa Lewis of safe additives and ones that should be avoided:

- *Food additives that seem to be SAFE*: acacia gum, adenosine 5 (avoid if on yeast-free diet), adipic acid, caseinates (avoid in a casein-free diet), ammonium salt compounds, annatto color (avoided by *some* celiacs), ascorbic acid, ascorbyl palmitate, beta carotene (avoid on "white diets"), calcium ascorbate (phosphate, salts, and sulfate), carbonates, cellulose gel/gum, disodium inosinate (avoid in yeast-free diets), EDTA, fumaric acid, gelatin, glycerides, lactic acid (avoid if *very* sensitive to dairy), lecithin (avoid if soy is a problem), pectin, potassium chloride (citrate, phosphate, sorbate), psyllium, and xanthan gum.
- *Food additives that should be AVOIDED*: all aluminum compounds, artificial colors, artificial flavors, aspartame (Nutrasweet), BHA, BHT, caffeine, calcium disodium EDTA, FD&C colors, monosodium glutamate (MSG), nitrates, nitrites, phosphoric acid, potassium bromate, quinine, olestra, polysorbate 60 (and 80), saccharin, sulfites, vanillin, TBHQ.

Further Reading for Healthier Eating

Rich Food, Poor Food: The Ultimate Grocery Purchasing System (GPS)

This detailed book by Jayson Calton, PhD, and Mira Calton, CN, can put our children on the path towards healthier eating. It offers a unique guide to steer us through the grocery store aisles. We can learn how to easily identify "rich foods" that are high in micronutrients, enhancing the health of our children. We can also learn how to avoid 150 "poor foods" that are lacking in micronutrients and can impede the health of our children. The book also discusses food ingredients commonly found in the United States that are banned in other countries. The authors identified thirteen of the worst ones and have graciously allowed us to share them with you in the table below. *Rich Food, Poor Food* can also teach us how to identify other potentially problematic ingredients we discussed in the food chapter including hormones, pesticides, and GMOs while helping us save money along the way. The authors have provided the following link to download the first three chapter of the book for free: https://caltonnutrition.leadpages.co/rich-food-poor-food. More information can be found on their website at www.caltonnutrition.com.

Some U.S. "Bad Boy" Ingredients Banned in Other Countries

Ingredient	Found in	Health Hazards
Arsenic	Poultry	Inorganic arsenic is classified by the EPA as a "human carcinogen"
Azodicarbonamide	Breads, frozen dinners, and packaged baked goods	Linked to asthma
BHA and BHT	Gum, nuts, butter, meat, and breakfast cereal	BHA may be a human carcinogen, a cancer-causing agent
Brominated vegetable oil (aka BVO)	Sports drinks and some citrus-flavored sodas	Competes with iodine for receptor sites in the body, which can lead to hypothyroidism, autoimmune disease, and thyroid cancer. The main ingredient, bromine, is a poisonous, corrosive chemical, linked to major organ system damage, birth defects, growth problems, schizophrenia, and hearing loss
Coloring agents: blue 1, blue 2, yellow 5, and yellow 6	Cake, candy, macaroni and cheese, medicines, sport drinks, soda, pet food, and cheese	Most artificial colors are made from coal tar, which is a carcinogen. Artificial food colors are also linked to hyperactivity and behavioral problems.
Olestra (aka Olean)	Fat-free potato chips	Depletion of fat-soluble vitamins and carotenoids. Side effects include severe gastrointestinal disturbances
Potassium bromate (aka brominated flour)	Rolls, wraps, bread crumbs, flatbread, chips	See bromine above. Associated with kidney and nervous system disorders, gastrointestinal discomfort
Synthetic hormones: rBGH and rBST	Milk and dairy products	Linked to breast, colon, and prostate cancers because it is supercharged with insulin growth factor-1

Courtesy of Jayson Calton, Mira Calton, and Mark Sisson, *Rich Food, Poor Food: The Ultimate Grocery Purchasing System (GPS)* (Malibu, CA: Primal Blueprint Pub., 2013).

The Unhealthy Truth

Written by Robyn O'Brien. Her first-person inspirational story was published in May 2009 by Random House, and reveals the alarming relationship between changes in our food and both the increase in dangerous allergies in our children and the increase in cancers in our families. Robyn's journey began when her daughter had a violent allergic reaction to eggs. She reveals all she uncovered and how she took on the food system, and offers a road map to healthy living. The Unhealthy Truth is a call to action that outlines how to keep our families safe. More information and helpful food resources can be found on Robyn's website at www.robynobrien.com. You can also check out her Ted Talk, "Patriotism on a Plate," on YouTube.

Consumer Organizations with Tools to Help Choose Healthy Food

GoodGuide

Their website enables consumers to retrieve health ratings on food and other consumer products such as personal care products, household products, and babies' and kids' products (phone apps available). It is convenient and easy. According to their website:

> GoodGuide's mission is to provide consumers with the information they need to make better shopping decisions. We believe that as more consumers choose products that contain ingredients with fewer health concerns, retailers and manufacturers face compelling incentives to make and sell better products. To fulfill our mission, GoodGuide combines manufacturer-provided information about product ingredients with authoritative information on the health effects of chemicals. We rate products so that consumers can have instant access to credible information about products that would be very difficult for anyone to develop on their own. We are a team of scientific experts in product and chemical information and have been engaged in this project for ten years. GoodGuide has grown to become the web's most comprehensive and credible resource for information about the impact of consumer products on human health. More than 1 million consumers use GoodGuide's website and mobile apps every month to help decode product labels, research ingredients, and make more informed decisions about the products they purchase.
>
> With GoodGuide, you can:
> - Use ratings to quickly identify the highest rated products on the market.
> - Find out whether a product contains ingredients with health concerns.
> - Rely on science expertise to interpret complex information about the potential health effects of different chemicals.
> - Get advice while shopping by using the GoodGuide iOS App, Product Scanner for Android, or the mobile website.

When we know what's in our food and household products, we can make better choices. If the millions of mothers out there shopping with a cell phone used this tool to influence their purchases, companies would have no choice but to respond with healthier products! You can find the GoodGuide at www.goodguide.com.

The Environmental Working Group (EWG)

The EWG has many food-related consumer product databases, just visit www.ewg.org and click on "consumer guides" for all the options below and more.

- EWG's Food Scores: This guide provides ratings of more than 80,000 products to help consumers make healthier, greener food choices. You can even take it with you to the grocery store when you download the mobile apps available.
- EWG's Dirty Dozen Guide to Food Additives: Here you will find a list of twelve additives that the EWG calls the "Dirty Dozen." They will tell you why, which foods contain them, and what you can do to avoid them.
- EWG's Shopper's Guide to Pesticides in Produce: This guide is updated yearly and annually ranks pesticide contamination on 48 popular fruits and vegetables, based on an analysis of more than 28,000 samples tested by the U.S. Department of Agriculture (USDA) and federal Food and Drug Administration (FDA). The Dirty Dozen and Clean Fifteen lists in the guide are based on these yearly pesticide residue tests. The guide can be downloaded to your phone for convenient shopping.
- The EWG also offers a Seafood Guide, Good Food on a Tight Budget Guide, and lots of GMO information.

GMO Resources

Non-GMO Shopping Guides

Below are shopping guide links to help you avoid GMOs. The links for *mobile phone apps* are available on the respective websites.

- The Non-GMO Shopping Guide, courtesy of the Institute for Responsible Technology and the Non-GMO Project, can be downloaded at www.NonGMOShoppingGuide.com.
- The GMO food list below is courtesy of the Institute for Responsible Technology (IRT). It includes some of the foods that may contain GM ingredients. Check out the IRT's free shopping guide above for additional details.
  - Infant formula
  - Salad dressing
  - Bread
  - Cereal
  - Hamburgers and hotdogs
  - Margarine
  - Mayonnaise
  - Crackers
  - Cookies
  - Chocolate
  - Candy
  - Fried food
  - Chips
  - Veggie burgers
  - Meat substitutes
  - Ice cream
  - Frozen yogurt
  - Tofu
  - Tamari and soy sauce
  - Soy cheese
  - Tomato sauce
  - Protein powder
  - Baking powder

- ° Any sugar not 100% cane
- ° Confectioner's glaze
- ° Alcohol
- ° Vanilla (may contain corn syrup)
- ° Peanut butter
- ° Enriched flour
- ° Pasta
- ° Malt
- ° White vinegar

GMO Labeling Efforts across the Country

The Center for Food Safety (CFS)

The CFS has been on the front lines fighting for GMO labeling laws and other important food safety legislation. The CFS website will provide you with the most up-to-date information on state and federal labeling initiatives. The site can also direct you to many resources including leaders in your area who are working to get GMO labeling laws passed. The True Food Network is their grassroots action network. Here you can sign up for updates and alerts including ways we can say no to industrialized food and demand true food. According to their website, "CFS is a national nonprofit, public interest, and environmental advocacy organization working to protect human health and the environment by curbing the use of harmful food production technologies and by promoting organic and other forms of sustainable agriculture." For the CFS website, go to www.centerforfoodsafety.org.

Local and State GMO Labeling Initiatives

Information on local and state GMO labeling efforts can be found at www.gefoodlabels.org/gmo-labeling/state-and-local-labeling-initiatives.

Label GMOs

This is the website for the original grassroots labeling initiative that started in California by a grandmother, Pamm Larry. This website contains great resources and media products to help spread the word! The Label GMOs website address is www.labelgmos.org.

Organic Consumer Association (OCA)

The OCA is committed to getting foods labeled and is a good resource for action. According to their website, "OCA is an online and grassroots nonprofit organization, the OCA also campaigns for health, justice, and sustainability. The OCA deals with crucial issues of food safety, industrial agriculture, genetic engineering, children's health, corporate accountability, Fair Trade, environmental sustainability, and other key topics. They are the only organization in the United States focused exclusively on promoting the views and interests of the nation's estimated 50 million organic and socially responsible consumers." You can visit the OCA website at www.organicconsumers.org.

Efforts to Boycott Companies Supporting GMOs

If you are interested in boycotting the companies (and all of their brands) who financially backed the defeat of GMO labeling legislation, visit the Organic Consumers Association (OCA) website discussed above. Here is the direct link to more information on the companies and the boycott guide: www.organicconsumers.org/news/comprehensive-boycott-guide.

Organizations Dedicated to Health Risks Associated with GMOs

Institute for Responsible Technology (IRT)
The IRT website by far offers the most comprehensive and up-to-date information on the science and health risks of GMOs including videos, podcasts, blogs, and reports. Everything on this site is well referenced, so you see the science (and links to study sources) behind the information. The IRT helped create the aforementioned Non-GMO Shopping Guide (also available to download free on their website) and allowed us to present the sample list of GMO foods in this guide. According to their website, "The IRT is a world leader in educating policymakers and the public about genetically modified (GM) foods and crops." IRT founder Jeffrey Smith is credited with "improving government policies and influencing consumer-buying habits." Smith authored the books *Seeds of Deception* and *Genetic Roulette*. In 2012, Smith directed and produced *Genetic Roulette*, a documentary film about GMOs that is narrated by Lisa Oz. This film provides compelling evidence about the harmful effects of GMOs and their possible role in many health problems in our children. A wealth of information on GMOs can be obtained from both the IRT website (www.responsibletechnology.org) and the website of the Non-GMO Project (www. nongmoproject.org) they sponsor.

Moms Across America
The growing grassroots organization Moms Across America educates the public about the dangers of GMOs and pesticides, including the damaging health effects they have on our children. Their website includes video interviews with doctors concerned about the health risks of GMOs to children and some great testimonials from mothers about the health improvements their children experienced after becoming GMO-free. Additional study information, articles, and reports are available. The Moms Across America website address is www.momsacrossamerica.com.

Sustainable Farming Information
Sustainable Table is a food program of Grace Communications Foundation. According to the Sustainable Table website, it "celebrates local sustainable food, educates consumers about the benefits of sustainable agriculture, and works to build community through food." Their website allows you to explore the issues surrounding sustainable food and agriculture; find out how to shop for and prepare sustainable food in the kitchen; take action and educate others; better understand factory farming through their award-winning online film *The Meatrix*; find farm stores, restaurants, CSAs, and other sustainable food sources in your area; and even understand the differences in food labels (all natural, organic, low fat, fat-free, etc.). This information and much more can be found on the website of Sustainable Table and Grace Communications at www.gracelinks.org.

Seafood Supplement

Fish Farming
- Fish sold in the United States are becoming more commonly raised in crowded aquafarms that also rely on antibiotics and other chemicals to produce fish at cheaper costs and higher profits—similar to factory farming of land animals.
- More than 90 percent of the shrimp and 70 percent of the salmon consumed in the United States are imported from areas that often use questionable fish farming methods, in which large quantities of shrimp and other fish are grown in cages, nets, and ponds with the use of antibiotics, hormones, and pesticides.
- Just like factory farm animals, fish are living in crowded and unnatural conditions that can become a breeding ground for diseases, parasitic infections, and debilitating injuries.

- These industrialized aquafarm facilities pose health threats to humans and the environment, and are rapidly replacing natural methods of fishing that have been used for ages.
- Considering that less than 2 percent of U.S. imported seafood is inspected, the best approach to avoid eating fish raised in an industrialized aquafarm facility is to know where your seafood comes from. Instead of eating imported farmed shrimp or salmon, consumers should look for shrimp or salmon caught wild or sustainably farmed in the United States. Sustainable fish farms do not pollute the environment with waste and use little or no wild fish in feed.

Fish Health Risks: Mercury and PCBs

- Fish commonly contain mercury and PCBs, which can pose serious health risks to everyone who consumes fish—not just children and pregnant woman. Please see below for a fish guide from the Environmental Defense Fund that lists the fish that often contain mercury and PCBs along with suggested maximum monthly intake levels.
- Fish and shellfish are an important part of a healthy diet. However, due to widespread contamination of fish with high levels of toxic mercury, health concerns for children and for pregnant and nursing women have surfaced.
- According to the FDA, some fish and shellfish contain high levels of mercury that may harm an unborn baby's or young child's developing nervous system. The FDA cites swordfish, shark, king mackerel, and tilefish as posing the greatest risk. The Environmental Working Group (EWG) researchers also cite tuna, sea bass, marlin, and halibut as being some of the worst contaminated fish.
- Both the FDA and the EPA make recommendations for pregnant women, nursing mothers, and children regarding fish consumption that includes avoiding fish with high levels of mercury and limiting weekly fish consumption. See fish advisory links for updated recommendations.
- Here's the problem we have with all of FDA and EPA recommendations . . . it has to do with the sum of the parts again. How do we know the existing levels of mercury in our body? There are many ways we can be exposed to mercury. A study by the EWG showed that 10 percent of U.S. women of childbearing age had high enough levels of mercury in their blood to already cause neurological harm to a fetus. Should we also be encouraged to explore alternative ways to get the nutrients fish can provide while pregnant or nursing?

Fish Advisories

- EPA/FDA: www.epa.gov/fish-tech/epa-fda-advisory-mercury-fish-and-shellfish.
- EWG: www.ewg.org/files/fishguide.pdf.
- Environmental Defense Fund (EDF): http://seafood.edf.org. Below is a general advisory for eating a few types of fish, courtesy of the EDF. A full list and updates are available on their website as well as additional information and a *sushi guide*.

Environmental Defense Fund Fish Advisory Chart

Maximum servings that can be safely eaten each MONTH*					
Fish Name	WOMEN	MEN	KIDS 6–12	KIDS 0–5	Health Risk
Swordfish	0	1	0	0	Mercury
Flounder (summer)	4+	4+	4+	4+	Mercury
Salmon, all varieties	4+	4+	4+	4+	Mercury
Tuna (light, canned)	4+	4+	4+	3	Mercury
Tuna (white albacore, canned)	3	3	2	1	Mercury
Tuna (big eye)	4	4	4	4	Unknown
Tuna (bluefin)	1	1	<1	<1	Mercury, PCBs
Striped bass (wild)	3	3	2	1	Mercury, PCBs
Striped bass (farmed)	4+	4+	4+	4+	Mercury
Grouper (imported)	2	2	1	1	Mercury
Black or red grouper (U.S. Gulf of Mexico)	2	2	1	1	Mercury
Crab (blue, red, dungeness, or king)	4+	4+	4+	4+	Mercury
Crab (U.S. snow)	4+	4+	4	4	Mercury
Cod (Alaska, U.S., Canada Pacific)	4+	4+	4+	4	Mercury
Halibut (Atlantic or Pacific)	4+	4+	3	2	Mercury
Tilapia	4+	4+	4+	4+	Mercury
Sea bass (black)	4	4	4	4	Mercury
Scallops	4+	4+	4+	4+	Mercury
Mahi-mahi	4+	4+	4+	3	Mercury
Shrimp	4+	4+	4+	4+	Mercury
Lobster (U.S., Maine)	4+	4+	4+	3	Mercury
Rainbow trout	4+	4+	4+	4+	Mercury

*[Authors' note: *Assuming no other contaminated fish is consumed. All references for the seafood supplement are included in the food chapter references.]*

Environmental Medicine

American Academy of Environmental Medicine (AAEM)
The website of the AAEM (www.aaemonline.org) can help you can locate a doctor in your area practicing environmental medicine. They also have posted on their website (under the Quick Links tab) their position statements, which provide an overview of their organization's philosophy.

In particular, a paper titled "An Overview of the Philosophy of the Environmental Medicine" written by Gary R. Oberg, MD, FAAEM, explains the basics of environmental medicine and how its unique approach may provide additional help and answers to many suffering from chronic health problems. This paper was written with healthcare providers in mind, but is easy to read and understand.

Environmental Medicine Books by Doris J. Rapp, MD
- Is This Your Child?
- Is This Your Child's World?
- Our Toxic World: A Wake Up Call
- 32 Tips That Could Save Your Life

Doris J. Rapp, MD, is a board-certified environmental medical specialist and pediatric allergist. She is also a *New York Times* best-selling author. Her first book—*Is This Your Child?*—describes the impact of food on children's behavior as well as their GI health. It helps parents identify common foods, chemicals, and allergic substances that could be causing behavior problems in your child or your child to be sick or feel unwell. This book includes mini case studies describing various health problems encountered by children and adults and the various environmental exposures that ended up being the root cause. The book *Our Toxic World: A Wake Up Call* discusses many chemical insults impacting our children's health (including food) and discusses ways you can prevent them. And her latest book, *32 Tips That Could Save Your Life,* may help you figure out exactly what it is that is making you sick, so you can better address the problem. More information on environmental factors affecting the health of both children and adults is available at www.drrapp.com.

Special Diets for Special Kids (volumes 1 and 2) by Dr. Lisa Lewis
Dr. Lewis's books are comprehensive, easy-to-read, and must-haves if you have a child with medical conditions. It includes many recipes as well as simplified scientific research supporting the connections between nutrition and a variety of childhood diseases and disorders. Specific nutritional advice is provided for various health conditions, and many hopeful stories are shared about how simply changing a diet can improve common health problems in children.

Resources for Chapter 6: Vaccines and Mental Health

Vaccine Ingredients
The sampling of some vaccine ingredients listed in this section were obtained from various manufacturers' product inserts.

Human and Animal Tissue
The manufacturing processes of many vaccines require growing viruses in human and animal tissue. FDA regulations require that any tissue used in the vaccine manufacturing process be screened for all known infectious diseases. However, there will always be health concerns about the potential for cross-contamination—a virus and/or disease in the living tissues being transferred into the vaccine a child receives.

Human blood proteins • Human lung cells • Human fetal lung cells • Human cell lines derived from aborted fetuses • Cow serum • Cow heart-muscle extract • Cow tissue extract • Monkey kidney cells • Guinea pig embryo cells • Chicken embryos • Chicken kidney cells • Chicken eggs

Antigens and Preservatives

All vaccines contain some form of antigens. This is what makes the vaccine work and stimulates the body to create an immune response to protect itself against a specific infection. Preservatives are used to prevent microbial contamination of the vaccine and are required for vaccines contained in multidose vials. Below are some common vaccine antigens and preservatives.

Live viruses • Inactivated viruses • Partial viruses • Partial bacteria •
Phenol • Thimerosal (mercury) • 2 phenoxyethanol (2-PE)

Adjuvants and Additives

Adjuvants are used to help the body create a better immune response to the vaccines. Additives are used to stabilize vaccine contents from adverse conditions such as heat or freeze-drying and from separating or sticking to the vial.

Aluminum salts • Fetal bovine (calf) serum • Monosodium glutamate (MSG) • Porcine (pig)
gelatin • Human serum albumin • Ammonium sulfate •
Egg proteins • Yeast • Sodium borate • Polysorbate 80 • Hydrochloric acid • Potassium chloride

Antibiotics and Inactivating Chemicals

Antibiotics are used to prevent bacterial contamination during the vaccine manufacturing process. Inactivating chemicals are critical components to vaccines because they kill the unwanted bacteria and inactivate infectious viruses used in the vaccines. For example, formaldehyde is used to inactivate the polio virus.

Neomycin • Streptomycin sulfate • Formadehyde • Gutaraldehyde

If you want to see the potential health effects from various chemicals noted in this section (or any chemical at all) a good resource to use is *The Good Guide Scorecard*. Scorecard integrates data from a large number of scientific and regulatory sources. Look for the Health Hazards tab to locate chemical profiles and their health effects. More information can be found at http://scorecard. goodguide.com.

Additional information on vaccine ingredients can be found at the following CDC website www.cdc.gov/vaccines/vac-gen/additives.htm.

Aluminum Supplement

FDA Regulations for Injected Aluminum Products vs. Vaccines

All forms of injectable aluminum contained in medicine products are required to have a warning label that says, "This product contains aluminum that may be toxic."

According to the code of federal regulations (21CFR201.323) surrounding labeling requirements for aluminum in large and small volume parenterals uses in total parenteral nutrition (IV feeding solution) and intravenous dextrose solution (sugar solution added to hospital IVs for hydration purposes) the following must appear in the labeling requirements:

> WARNING: This product contains aluminum that may be toxic. Aluminum may reach toxic levels with prolonged parenteral administration if kidney function is impaired. Premature neonates are particularly at risk because their kidneys are immature, and they require large amounts of calcium and phosphate solutions, which contain aluminum.
>
> Research indicates that patients with impaired kidney function, including premature neonates, who receive parenteral levels of aluminum at greater than 4 to 5

[micro]g/kg/day accumulate aluminum at levels associated with central nervous system and bone toxicity. Tissue loading may occur at even lower rates of administration.

The FDA also limits the amount of injected aluminum medicine can contain and the following is required in the labeling: "Drug product contains no more than 25 mcg/L [micrograms per liter] of aluminum."

Just to give you an idea of how much injected aluminum people receive . . . while hospitalized an adult will typically get about one liter of intravenous feeding solution a day, equating to 25 mcg of injected aluminum. At birth a newborn is recommended to receive the hepatitis B immunization, containing 250 mcg of aluminum. At the two-month visit they could exceed 1,000 mcg of aluminum as they could be subjected to multiple vaccines containing aluminum in a single visit (hep B booster, Hib, and DTaP).

The warning label quoted above discusses aluminum toxicity concerns notably for premature babies when levels exceed 4 to 5 mcg per kilogram of body weight per day. When trying to equate this safety standard to the body weight of a newborn for "general comparison" it equates to not exceeding 20 mcg of aluminum for an 8-pound baby. Yet, our vaccine schedule suggests giving newborn babies a hepatitis B immunization that contains 250 mcg of aluminum. Does the difference between a neonate (preemie) and newborn warrant exceeding safety guidelines more than 10 times over?

[Authors' note: Weight conversions are as follows 8 pounds is 3.6 kg (rounded up is 4 kg). The FDA suggests limiting aluminum to 5 mcg of aluminum per every kg of weight equating to a 20 mcg limit for an 8-pound infant.]

FDA Vaccine Regulation Regarding Injected Aluminum

The FDA does have a federal regulation (21CFR610.15) regarding the aluminum content in vaccines. The FDA "limits" the amount of aluminum in each single vaccine dose to between 0.85 mg and 1.25 mg which is actually 850 mcg–1,250 mcg—that's how much aluminum a single dose of vaccine is actually permitted to contain. That's many times over the safety limits set for other injectable aluminum products (one is set at 25 mcg/L/day and one is set at 5 mcg/ per kg body weight/day). Where is the common sense in a vaccine safety guideline that permits infants and children to receive much, much higher amounts of aluminum than would be permitted in other injectable aluminum products?

How Much Aluminum Is in Childhood Vaccines?

Hib (PedVaxHib brand only): 225 mcg

Hepatitis B: 250 mcg.

DTaP: depending on the manufacturer, ranges from 170 to 625 mcg

Pneumococcus (Pc): 125 mcg

Hepatitis A: 250 mcg

HPV: 225 mcg to 500 mcg

Pentacel (DTaP, HIB and Polio combo vaccine): 330 mcg

Pediarix (DTaP, Hep B and Polio combo vaccine): 850 mcg

[Authors' note: All references for the aluminum supplement—including the regulatory documents regarding injected aluminum—can be found in the Chapter 6 references.]

More Reading on Aluminum

For more information on this topic we suggest *The Vaccine Book: Making the Right Decision for Your Child* by Bob Sears, MD, FAAP, a board-certified pediatrician. The book is part of the best-selling Sears parenting library and contains much more detailed information about aluminum toxicity studies (and much more on vaccines). The book is easy to read. In our opinion it is very fair and balanced. It is not an antivaccine book. It does however discuss what some may consider to be a controversial topic: alternate vaccine schedules. While some may find this controversial, many others find this a very helpful solution when vaccinating, especially those who have safety concerns about the current schedule. Some of the aluminum information contained in *The Vaccine Book* has been posted on Dr. Bob's website at www.askdrsears.com. The aluminum information can be located on the website by following the links for Health Concerns, Vaccines, and finally Vaccine FAQs.

Manufacturer's Package Inserts

The most complete and reliable source of information available to us on any vaccination can be found in the manufacturer's package insert for each separate vaccine. We encourage you to read these before vaccinating. Full prescribing inserts will contain important information regarding drug interactions, contraindications, adverse reactions, warnings, precautions, ingredients, and effectiveness. Vaccine package inserts should be made available to view wherever your child receives their vaccinations, and all package inserts for vaccines approved for use can be found on the FDA website at www.fda.gov/BiologicsBloodVaccines/Vaccines/ApprovedProducts/ucm093833.htm.

Once on the above FDA site, click on the specific vaccine (listed by manufacturers) you are looking for. You will then be redirected to a new page for that particular manufacturer's vaccine and related information. On this page you will need to find the link for the package insert.

The Institute for Vaccine Safety at Johns Hopkins
Bloomberg School of Public Health

This website also allows you to access manufacturers' product inserts. According to their website, the Institute for Vaccine Safety was established in 1997 at the Johns Hopkins University School of Public Health—now the Johns Hopkins Bloomberg School of Public Health. Their mission is "to provide an independent assessment of vaccines and vaccine safety to help guide decision makers and educate physicians, the public, and the media about key issues surrounding the safety of vaccines. The Institute's goal is to work toward preventing disease using the safest vaccines possible." The Institute supports vaccination of all children with all government recommended vaccines. Their website is www.vaccinesafety.edu.

The National Vaccine Information Center (NVIC)

The NVIC website is another way you can access manufacturers' product inserts. Under "diseases and vaccines," each separate disease will give you access to the related vaccine manufacturer's product inserts. According to their website,

> The NVIC is a national charitable, nonprofit educational organization founded in 1982. NVIC launched the vaccine safety and informed consent movement in America in the early 1980s and is the oldest and largest consumer-led organization advocating for the institution of vaccine safety and informed consent protections in the public health system. The NVIC is dedicated to the prevention of vaccine injuries and deaths through public education and to defending the informed consent ethic in medicine. As an independent clearinghouse for information on diseases and vaccines, NVIC does not advocate for or against the use of vaccines. The NVIC supports the availability of all preventive healthcare options, including vaccines, and the right of consumers to make educated, voluntary healthcare choices.

The NVIC website address is www.nvic.org.

Reporting a Vaccine Reaction (VAERS)

According to the VAERS website, "VAERS is a national vaccine safety surveillance program co-sponsored by the Centers for Disease Control and Prevention (CDC) and the Food and Drug Administration (FDA). VAERS is a post-marketing safety surveillance program that collects information about adverse events (possible side effects) that occur after the administration of vaccines licensed for use in the United States."

If you suspect that you or your child has experienced a vaccine reaction, you are encouraged to report that reaction *yourself* to the government through the Vaccine Adverse Event Reporting System (VAERS). Reporting a potential vaccine reaction helps researchers improve vaccine safety for our children. Since 1990, the U.S. government has collected reports of adverse health events that follow the administration of vaccinations. You can access VAERS at the following web address for more information: www.vaers.hhs.gov.

Searching the VAERS Database for Vaccine Reaction Information

CDC Wonder is the U.S. government's official search engine where you can access the VAERS database. It is a menu-driven system that is easy to use. A video demonstration is available providing information on how to search the VAERS database using CDC Wonder and also explains the purpose of VAERS and the strengths and limits of the VAERS data. The VAERS data can be searched in a variety of ways and can be accessed at https://wonder.cdc.gov/vaers.html.

The National Vaccine Information Center (NVIC) hosts MedAlerts, the very first online search engine that gave the public an easy-to-use tool to review and analyze VAERS data (before CDC Wonder). Many find this site to be more user-friendly, with more extensive reporting capabilities and more powerful search capabilities. MedAlerts allows users to search and review reports of vaccine-related complications made to the federal VAERS. It allows the VAERS database to be searched for reported adverse events in a variety of ways such as by symptoms of reactions, state of residence, age, gender, disease, vaccine, manufacturer, dates and more. You can access MedAlerts at www.medalerts.org.

Vaccine Injury Table Listing Vaccine Reactions

The Vaccine Injury Table provided online by the U.S. Department of Health and Human Services Health Resources and Services Administration (HRSA) makes it easier to know if it is possible to get compensation due to a vaccine injury. Although most people will not have a serious problem following vaccinations, the HRSA table lists and explains injuries/conditions that are presumed to be caused by vaccines along with the time periods in which the first symptom of these injuries/conditions must occur after receiving the vaccine in order to eligible. The table of presumed vaccine-related injuries that may be eligible for compensation can be found at www.hrsa.gov/vaccinecompensation/vaccinetable.html.

Other Vaccine Topics

Vaccine State Laws

Information on state-by-state vaccine legislation can be found on the website of the Institute for Vaccine Safety at Johns Hopkins Bloomberg School of Public Health. This site also provides a great visual map showing each U.S. state and which vaccine exemptions are available in that state and offers many other valuable vaccine resources. You can visit the map of state exemptions at www.vaccinesafety.edu/cc-exem.htm.

Additionally, if you are interested in protecting your right to choose vaccinations, you can find ways to exercise your voice at the NVIC website. You will also find lots of information on past and current legislation related to vaccines. You can access this information through their Advocacy Portal located at https://nvicadvocacy.org/members/Home.aspx.

The Vaccine Ingredients Calculator
A valuable tool provided by the National Vaccine Information Center, the vaccine calculator can save you time researching ingredients and brand choices. It allows you to view all available manufacturer brands for any vaccines on the recommended schedule, provides a list of ingredients in each brand for easy comparison, and also allows you to examine just how much aluminum, thimerosal, and other ingredients are contained in the various vaccines (if any). By walking through the vaccinations your child is scheduled to receive, you can develop a personalized plan and more readily discuss your preferred brand choices and any other concerns with your child's healthcare provider. To use this tool or to learn more about the Vaccine Ingredients Calculator visit the NVIC website at www.nvic.org. Information on the Vaccine Ingredients Calculator is located under the Vaccines tab. Here is the direct link to the calculator: www.vaccine-tlc.org.

Boosting the Immune System to Prevent Vaccine Reactions
Robert W. Sears, MD, FAAP, a board-certified pediatrician has posted an online article on the previously mentioned AskDrSears website. The article contains many additional details to the recommended suggestions in the vaccine chapter to boost your child's immune system prior to vaccinating. The article stems from his best-selling vaccine book titled *The Vaccine Book: Making the Right Decision for Your Child.*
The article can be accessed at Dr. Sears's Website, www.AskDrSears.com.
Once on this site go to the Health Concerns tab and click on Vaccines. The article is one of the vaccine articles posted at the bottom of the page. AskDrSears.com has a wealth of information intended to help parents become better-informed consumers of healthcare and includes many valuable vaccine resources.

Finding a Doctor Who Supports Vaccine Choice
To provide assistance to those living in states with laws that facilitate choosing to delay vaccines or decline vaccinations the AskDrSears website provides a list of doctors who are "vaccine friendly" and willing to work with your personal choice. The article "Find a Vaccine-Friendly Doctor Near You" can be accessed at www.AskDrSears.com. Additional articles are available concerning alternative vaccine schedules. Once on this site go to the Health Concerns tab and click on Vaccines. Once you are on the vaccine page, these vaccine articles are posted at the bottom. You can also find support and additional resources at NVIC.org.

Vaccine Documentary Mini-Series

The Truth About Vaccines
This comprehensive 7-episode documentary series brings together 60 health experts from around the world to discuss both sides of the vaccine debate including: the history of vaccines, vaccine risks and safety concerns, vaccine options and alternatives. This series is dedicated to bringing you the facts so you can make your own informed decision. It goes deeper into all the topics discussed in the vaccine chapter and hits on some new topics as well. Filmmaker, NY Times Bestselling Author, parent, and health freedom advocate, Ty Bollinger, is your host. More information can be found at go.thetruthaboutvaccines.com.

Mental Health Resources

The Substance Abuse and Mental Health Services Administration
The Substance Abuse and Mental Health Services Administration (SAMHSA) is an agency within the U.S. Department of Health and Human Services that, according to their website, "leads public

health efforts to advance the behavioral health of the nation. SAMHSA's mission is to reduce the impact of substance abuse and mental illness on America's communities."

The SAMHSA website is a great place to start when looking for up-to-date evidence-based mental health research, treatment, and services. Information on this site includes both drug-free behavioral interventions and medication-based behavioral interventions. This site offers help to anyone looking to access treatments and services. Look for the children's tab for child-specific behavioral health treatment services. The site provides a *treatment locator* where you can simply enter your zip code and find mental health/behavioral health services in your community. And also offers 24-hour, toll-free hotlines to answer questions and provide help in a crisis. The SAMHSA website address is www.samhsa.gov.

The National Resource Center on ADHD
The National Resource Center on ADHD is the national clearinghouse for the latest evidence-based information on ADHD. The program is sponsored by CHADD (Children and Adults with Attention Deficit/Hyperactivity Disorder) and is supported by the CDC. According to the CDC, "the Center provides comprehensive information and support to individuals with ADHD, their families and friends, and the professionals involved in their lives." More information can be found on their website www.help4adhd.org.

Information on Psychiatric Drugs and Potential Side Effects
Once again, manufacturers' product inserts will provide you with the most detailed and complete information on any drug your child takes including its approved uses, contradictions, side effects, ingredients, and warnings. All manufacturers' product inserts can be accessed on the website of DailyMed. They are the official provider of FDA label information or package inserts for marketed drugs. The site is provided by the National Library of Medicine as a public service. According to the DailyMed website, they "provide a standard, comprehensive, up-to-date, look-up and download resource of medication content and labeling found in medication package inserts." Visit the DailyMed website at www.dailymed.nlm.nih.gov/dailymed/index.cfm.

Online Psychiatric Drug Search Engine
This search engine is sponsored by the Citizens Commission on Human Rights (CCHR), a mental health watchdog group, and provides information on psychiatric drug side effects. This online tool gives a summary of three different sources of data on documented psychiatric drug risks, including:

• International drug regulatory warnings
• Studies published in worldwide medical journals
• Adverse reaction reports filed with the U.S. Food and Drug Administration between 2004 and 2012 by doctors, pharmacists, healthcare providers, attorneys, and consumers.

CCHR presents the downside of psychiatric drug therapy—the documented risks—and also provides valuable information on drug-free alternatives to mental health disorders. The psychiatric drug search engine can be accessed on the CCHR website: www.cchrint.org/psychdrugdangers

[Authors' note: Please know that the information on the CCHR site is clearly antidrug therapy and will not offer balanced information that may include benefits of drug therapy.]

Further Reading and Solutions for Mental Health Problems in Children
Author Scott M. Shannon, MD, is assistant clinical professor of psychiatry at the University of Colorado and past president of the American Board of Integrative Holistic Medicine. Dr. Shannon is board-certified in child/adolescent psychiatry and integrative holistic medicine. He teaches healthcare professionals around the world how to approach children's health and well-being

holistically. He is the founder of the Wholeness Center in Fort Collins, Colorado, the largest and most comprehensive integrative mental health clinic in the United States, and is the founder of the Integrative Psychiatric Intensive Program, an innovative, focused program for holistic mental health. Below are highly recommended books he has written to help parents (and teachers) find holistic solutions to behavioral health challenges facing many of today's children.

Mental Health for the Whole Child by Scott Shannon, MD: Every child possesses enormous untapped potential, and yet the number of kids suffering from mental illness today seems to creep ever upward. Depression, anxiety, ADHD, OCD, oppositional defiant disorder, anger issues—you name it—are increasingly prevalent, leaving clinician's offices packed with worried parents and caregivers, wondering how they can help their children. In this book, child psychiatrist Scott Shannon offers a refreshing new path for practitioners who are eager for a more optimistic view of children's mental health, one that emphasizes a child's inherent resilience and resources over pathology and prescriptions.

Parenting the Whole Child: A Holistic Child Psychiatrist Offers Practical Wisdom on Behavior, Brain Health, Nutrition, Exercise, Family Life, Peer Relationships, School Life, Trauma, Medication, and More by Scott Shannon, MD, with Emily Heckman: This book is meant as a parent's guide to Dr. Shannon's book for professionals *Mental Health for the Whole Child* noted above. In this book Scott Shannon equips parents and caregivers with a better way to understand the mental health challenges their children face, including how cutting-edge scientific concepts like epigenetics and neuroplasticity mean new hope for overcoming them. Readers learn how the most common stressors in kids—inadequate nutrition, unaddressed trauma, learning problems, family relationships, and more—are often at the root of behavioral and emotional issues, and what steps can be taken to restore health and wholeness, without immediately turning to medication.

Resources for Chapter 7: Environment

The Body Burden of Chemicals

The Environmental Working Group (EWG)
The EWG is one of our favorite organizations. According to their website, they are "A research and advocacy group focused on protecting human health and the environment." They also work tirelessly to influence laws so that the health of our children stands protected. We discussed their breakthrough research on chemicals found in umbilical cord blood at the opening of the environmental chapter. Below is more information on the study and the critically acclaimed video that highlights its results. Their website is overflowing with helpful resources, tips, and guides you can use right now to impact the health and safety your family: www.ewg.org.

Body Burden Studies and 10 Americans Video
This is one of the most powerful and eye-opening videos we have ever seen (about 20 minutes). EWG president Ken Cook presents to a live audience the results of their pioneering study about the chemical pollution found in newborns. It provides additional details that we only touched on in the opening of the environmental chapter. Watch this video and you will quickly understand the connection between the environment and our children's health. It can be viewed on the EWG website at www.ewg.org/news/videos/10-americans. The report was issued under the title *Body Burden: The Pollution in Newborns*.

Water Supplement

How Can We Protect Our Children's Drinking Water?

In addition to the steps below, that may cost money, one of the simplest and cheapest ways we can purify many contaminants from our water is by bringing it to a rolling boil on the stovetop for at least one minute.

Step 1: Find Out What Contaminants Are in Our Tap Water

Most convenient option: We can go to the EWG's National Drinking Water Database to find out if there are contaminants identified in our local drinking water that pose health concerns. It is as easy as plugging in our zip code. This extensive national database receives water contaminant data from public and environmental health agencies around the country that *may not* have shown up in our annual water quality report. EWG's National Drinking Water Database can be accessed at www.ewg.org/tap-water.

Most comprehensive option: We can have our drinking water tested independently. This option will cost us some time and some money ($150 and up for a good test). One drawback to this option is that we need to know *what* we want to test for. We need to identify what specific contaminants are of concern to us so our test is of value. These concerns will vary depending on where we live and what toxic chemicals are being released in our community by various industries (or natural sources) that could threaten our drinking water. The EWG's National Drinking Water Database noted above is a resource to find this information. Additionally, the EPA's Toxic Release Inventory (TRI) website is a great resource to help us identify toxic releases in our community. We can then use all this information as a springboard for our independent water tests. More detailed information on the EPA's TRI can be found in the next section. Check out EPA's TRI website at www2.epa.gov/toxics-release-inventory-tri-program.

Always an option: We can always contact our local water provider to get more detailed information on our local water testing and reports. But remember that our local water provider only has to test for contaminates that are federally regulated by the EPA, unless, of course, our state or our community have put more stringent controls in place.

Step 2: Get a Good Home Water Filtration System That Fits Our Specific Water Needs

Because water treatment plants are not equipped to remove all contaminants that may end up in our drinking water, many concerned parents use home filtration systems to further treat water from public supplies or wells. Water filtration systems are not all the same, and we should invest in one that filters out the specific contaminants we are concerned with. For example, carbon filters can filter out PFOA and PFOS, while a reverse osmosis water filter may be needed to remove a chemical contaminant such as hexavalent chromium (chromium 6). The EWG has an extensive online guide to help us find a home filtration system that fits our specific needs. The Food and Water Watch also offers help with finding a good water filtration system. More information is below under drinking-water resources.

Drinking-Water Resources

✓ Clean Water Action is a national citizen's organization of over one million members working for clean, safe, and affordable water, as well as prevention of health-threatening pollution. Lots of valuable resources and publications (oil and gas pollution, fracking, nuclear power plants, clean drinking water) are available on their website at www.cleanwateraction.org.

✓ EWG's National Drinking Water Database provides comprehensive information on drinking water in the United States. This is where you can find out if there are any contaminants of concern in your local drinking water by simply entering your zip code.

You can then use this information to spring board into ways to make your drinking water safer. Access the database at www.ewg.org/tap-water.

✓ EWG's Guide to Safe Drinking Water is available at www.ewg.org/research/ewgs-guide-safe-drinking-water.

✓ EWG's Water Filter Buying Guide answers all your home water filtration questions and helps guide you through buying a water filtration system that fits your needs. It's accessible at www.ewg.org/tap-water/getawaterfilter.php.

✓ Food and Water Watch provides extensive resources on our water at www.foodandwaterwatch.org

✓ EPA's Learn about Water homepage provides a wealth of information on drinking-water sources, safeguards in place to protect our drinking water, current drinking-water standards and risk management, water security, and many other resources we can tap into. It even includes information on where our local drinking-water sources originate from and ways we can get involved in protecting our local drinking-water sources. The EPA has set up a toll free safe drinking-water hotline (1-800-426-4791) to answer consumer questions related to drinking water (and groundwater) programs authorized under the Safe Drinking Water Act. The web address for the EPA's Water webpage is www.epa.gov/learn-issues/learn-about-water.

Toxic Pollution in Your Community

EPA's Toxic Release Inventory Program

Information on toxic chemical releases by industries in every community must be reported to the EPA's Toxic Release Inventory Program (TRI) and made public so citizens like us have access to this valuable environmental health information. The process is as simple as entering your zip code on an EPA website to find out which businesses are releasing toxins in your community, what those toxins are, what levels are being released, and what the possible health effects may be. It is an eye-opening experience and an incredible resource many are unaware of. Once you know what specific industrial chemicals are threatening your local drinking water, you can have an independent water test done to see if those specific contaminants are in your water *or* simply base your water filtration needs directly on these contaminants of concern. (Please note that some industries are exempt from reporting.) Access the inventory at www2.epa.gov/toxics-release-inventory-tri-program.

The GoodGuide

Just plug in your zip code to get a quick overview of many toxic releases in your community and a ranking of your local county against all others across the country to see how your community measures up with toxic releases, air and water quality, and even environmental justice. You can also find information on potential EPA Superfund sites in your area and the list of contaminates found at the site with action plans for remediation. You can find the GoodGuide at http://scorecard.goodguide.com.

View AIR Quality in Your Community

Finding out about your air quality is as simple as entering your zip code at the EPA's AIRNow website. According to their website, "The U.S. EPA, NOAA, NPS, tribal, state, and local agencies developed the AIRNow website to provide the public with easy access to national air quality information." AIRNow offers daily air quality forecasts and real-time air quality conditions for over 400 cities across the United States and provides links to more detailed state and local air quality and health information. The EPA's AIRNow website can be accessed at www.airnow.gov.

Chemicals of Concern

Safer Chemicals, Healthy Families

According to their website, "The Safer Chemicals, Healthy Families coalition represents more than 11 million individuals and includes parents, health professionals, advocates for people with learning disabilities, reproductive health advocates, environmentalists, and businesses from across the nation." They work together to safeguard our children from toxic chemicals in our homes, places of work, and products we use every day.

Here you can access much more information on their list of chemicals of concern that we presented in Chapter 7: BPA, formaldehyde, heavy metals (mercury, arsenic, and lead), hexane, hexavalent chromium, methylene chloride, PCBs and DDT, perfluorinated compounds, PBTs (persistent, bioaccumulative, and toxic chemicals), phthalates, toxic flame retardants (PBDEs, TDCP, TCEP), tricholoroethylene (TCE), and vinyl chloride. You can check out fact sheets on each of them that are based on leading peer-reviewed science. Their site also allows you to join the movement to push Congress and retailers for stronger action on toxic chemicals. Check out Safer Chemicals, Healthy Families at http://saferchemicals.org/get-the-facts/chemicals-of-concern.

Washington Toxics Coalition/Toxic-Free Future

According to their website, "After 35 years, the Washington Toxics Coalition became Toxic-Free Future to better represent the organization's hopeful vision for how the world should be for our families and environment. Our Mission: Toxic-Free Future advocates for the use of safer products, chemicals, and practices through advanced research, advocacy, grassroots organizing, and consumer engagement to ensure a healthier tomorrow. They helped establish strong new requirements in Washington state for makers of children's products to disclose harmful chemicals in their products. This is now the global standard for companies making kids' products that range from pacifiers and toys to cribs, car seats, and shampoos.

On their website homepage, look for the Science tab; here you can find Chemicals of Concern. Here you can get more detailed information on the following: Perfluorinated compounds (Teflon and stain protectors), toxin flame retardants, phthalates, pesticides, PCBs and DDT, heavy metals (mercury, lead, arsenic), formaldehyde, BPA, and antimony. Their website provides detailed information on each chemical or chemical family as well as additional information on ways we are exposed, why we should be concerned about the health risks, and ways we can protect ourselves from these toxins. Visit Toxic-Free Future at www.toxicfreefuture.org.

Hidden Toxins in the Home and School

Also, check out the Toxic-Free Future website for their Healthy Living, Healthy Kids, and Healthy Homes sections, full of tools and tips to keep your kids safe from toxic products in and around the home and school! These include a closer look at the nursery and playroom, toys and clothing, arts and crafts supplies, schools and daycares, indoor pest control, and more. They also have Healthy Pregnancy, Healthy Gardens, Healthy Bodies, and Healthy Food sections. Visit the Toxic-Free Future website at www.toxicfreefuture.org.

Consumer Product Databases

The GoodGuide

The site contains health evaluations on thousands of personal care, food, and household products. There is a separate "babies and kids" product category. GoodGuide's 0 to 10 rating system helps consumers quickly evaluate and compare consumer products based on their ingredients. Mobile phone apps are available. More detailed information was presented on the GoodGuide in the Food Resource Guide. Visit the GoodGuide website at www.goodguide.com.

Environmental Working Group (EWG)

The EWG has multiple consumer product databases; just visit www.ewg.org and click on consumer guides for the options described below and many more.

- EWG's Skin Deep Guide to Cosmetics: This is EWG's personal care products database, which includes much more than cosmetics. It rates over 80,000 personal care products and is the world's largest personal care product safety guide. Skin Deep's product ratings are based on the known hazards associated with ingredients listed on labels. It has a separate Babies and Moms product category.
- EWG's Guide to Healthy Cleaning: This is an interactive rating system that scores 2,000 popular cleaning products for toxicity and disclosure of contents. See how the products you use rate and possibly find healthier alternatives.
- EWG's Sunscreen Guide: This guide annually rates the safety and effectiveness of over 1,000 sunscreens, daily moisturizers, makeups, and lip products that have SPF values. According to EWG, they base their safety assessments on ingredients listed on product labels.
- EWG's Dirty Dozen of Endocrine Disruptors (Keep a Breast): This is a newer guide highlighting the most common and most harmful hormone-altering chemicals and how to avoid them.
- EWG's Healthy Child Healthy World Program: Dedicated to helping empower parents, drive solutions, and shape policy to protect children's health. We encourage you to watch the award-winning video *A Wake Up Story* to learn how to protect your family from everyday hazards impacting their health and join a movement to protect the health of all children (takes less than four minutes of your time to watch).

Household Products Database

The Household Products Database of the National Library of Medicine is based on the Consumer Product Information Database. It links products to health effects from material safety data sheets (MSDS) provided by manufacturers and allows consumers to research products based on chemical ingredients. Here is the link to the database: www.householdproducts.nlm.nih.gov.

More Consumer Resources

Mind the Store Campaign

Mind the Store Campaign of Safer Chemicals, Healthy Families invites you to join the national effort to tell retailers to get tough on toxic chemicals in consumer products. According to the Mind the Store website, they are "challenging major U.S. retailers to adopt policies to identify, restrict, and safely substitute the Hazardous 100+ chemicals in common consumer products." You can simply sign up for action alerts and, in less than a minute, make a difference by simply clicking a button to let a specific retailer know your desire for safer products. This campaign is making a difference to protect our families from toxic chemicals. Please visit Mind the Store for ways you can take action: www.mindthestore.org.

The Story of Stuff Project

The Story of Stuff Project is a highly recommended and highly acclaimed online tool where you can learn more about overconsumption and many other environmental and consumer issues through web films made by creator and author Annie Leonard. It's one of the most watched environmental video series of all time. *The Story of Stuff* film started it all. It is a powerful and funny twenty-minute film that exposes the connections between many of our current environmental and social issues by taking a closer look at our production and consumption patterns. You can also join the Story of Stuff Project community of half a million change makers worldwide working to build a healthier and just planet. Many additional great short environmental videos are available for viewing on The Story of Stuff Project website under the Resources tab. Visit www.storyofstuff.org.

Persistent, Bioaccumlative, Toxic Chemicals (PBTs)

Here is a partial list of PBTs, courtesy of Safer Chemicals, Healthy Families: anthracene, asbestos, cadmium and cadmium compounds chloroalkanes, C10-13 (short-chain chlorinated paraffins), p-Dichlorobenzene, hexabromobiphenyl, hexabromocyclododecane, hexachlorobutadiene, lead and lead compounds, mercury and mercury compounds, musk xylene, pentachlorobenzene, perfluorooctane sulfonic acid, perfluorooctane sulfonyl fluoride, phenanthrene, polybrominated biphenyls, polybrominated diphenylethers (PBDEs), polychlorinated terphenyls, tetrabromobisphenol A, 1,2,3-trichlorobenzene, 1,2,4-trichlorobenzene, 1,2,3,4-tetrachlorobenzene, and 1,2,4,5-tetrachlorobenzene. More information on PBTs can be found on the Safer Chemicals, Healthy Families website: www.saferchemicals.org.

Endocrine-Disrupting Hormones

The EWG and the Keep a Breast Foundation have provided the Dirty Dozen list of the 12 most common and most harmful hormone-altering chemicals and how to avoid them. The list can be found on the EWG website at www.ewg.org.

Plastics and PVC

The Center for Health, Environment, and Justice (CHEJ) offers safety recommendations including choosing nonplastic products whenever possible. If you do choose plastic products, be sure to avoid the recycling symbol labeled #3 or the initials PVC, which means it was used in that product. The following plastics may also have a negative effect on our children's health, so watch out for them as well: polycarbonate (PC, #7), polystyrene (PS, #6) and acrylonitrile butadiene styrene (ABS; this was not part of the original plastics ID system so it has no number).

The CHEJ website offers many valuable publications to protect our children's health, including a PVC publication with many resources, such as the "Back-to-School Guide to PVC-Free School Supplies." You can locate this guide under the Take Action tab on the CHEJ website at www.chej.org. Look for Publications (PVC).

According to their website, "CHEJ acts to build healthy communities nationwide, with social justice, economic well-being, and democratic governance. We provide essential resources, strategic partnerships, and training to local leaders to achieve this mission." Some additional campaigns of the CHEJ include Be Safe (a nationwide initiative to build support for the precautionary approach); Children's Environmental Health Program (a campaign to address issues such as safe school siting, nontoxic pest management, least toxic cleaning products and procedures, indoor air quality, and more); Prevent Fracking Harms (a campaign to increase awareness of harms from fracking, e.g., drinking-water contamination); and Focus on Schools (a program that provides resources for keeping school environments safe). Check out all CHEJ campaings at the Center for Health, Environment, and Justice website at www.chej.org.

Fracking

The Food and Water Watch website has additional on information on fracking and fossil fuels. You can join the movement to help ban fracking by signing the Food and Water Watch online petition. You can also learn how to work in your community to protect local food and water from fracking and other environmental insults. More information under the campaigns tab on the Food and Water Watch homepage at www.foodandwaterwatch.org.

Environmental Health Resources

The Collaborative on Health and the Environment (CHE)

According to their website, "The CHE is committed to protecting the health of families, children, and communities from pollution and other environmental factors that contribute to chronic disease and disability. By cultivating a diverse, dynamic, science-based learning community, CHE strengthens our collective capacity to translate the latest environmental health research into health-promoting programs, policies and practices." The CHE offers an initiative on children's environmental health, ScienceServ, that provides some great information and resources. According to their website, ScienceServ "explores the promotion of children's health through prevention of environmental exposures and other factors that undermine healthy development." You'll find more information on Children's Health ScienceServ, on the CHE website at www.healthandenvironment. org.

The National Institute of Environmental Health Sciences (NIEHS)

The NIEHS is part of the National Institutes of Health. NIEHS's broad focus on the environmental causes of disease makes the institute a unique part of NIH. According to their website, the mission of the NIEHS is "to discover how the environment affects people in order to promote healthier lives." NIEHS is home to the National Toxicology Program, the nation's premier program for testing and evaluation of agents in our environment. Some of the research areas being addressed at NIEHS include autism, air pollution and asthma, cancer, climate change and health, developmental basis of adult disease, nanomaterials, metal toxicity, endocrine disruptors, and pesticides. Kids Environment Kids Health is an NIEHS "resource for kids, parents, and teachers to find fun and educational materials related to health, science, and the environment we live in today." The NIEHS also publishes a monthly journal (discussed below). Visit the NIEHS website at www.niehs.nih.gov.

Environmental Health Perspectives (EHP)

This monthly journal of peer-reviewed research and news is published by the NIEHS. It is a top-ranked monthly journal in environmental sciences. All EHP content is free online at http://ehp. niehs.nih.gov.

The Children's Environmental Health Network (CEHN)

According to their website, CEHN "is a national multidisciplinary organization whose mission is to protect the developing child from environmental health hazards and promote a healthier environment." To achieve this mission, the network has several goals:

- to promote the development of sound public health and child-focused national policy
- to stimulate prevention-oriented research
- to educate health professionals, policymakers, and community members in preventive strategies
- to elevate public awareness of environmental hazards to children

The network also publishes many different resources on Children's Environmental Health. You can find more information on the CEHN website at www.cehn.org.

Environmental Health Free E-book

The Story of Health is a beautifully illustrated, multimedia book that simply and clearly explains multiple factors that influence our health across the lifespan through storytelling. It includes easy-to-understand information on our natural, built, chemical, food, economic, and social environments, as well as how these environments interact with each other and genetics. The e-book series includes fictional case stories including "Brett's Story" (asthma), "Stephen's Story" (cancer/childhood leukemia), and "Amelia's Story" (developmental disabilities).

The Story of Health was developed by the Agency for Toxic Substances and Disease Registry (ATSDR); the Collaborative on Health and the Environment (CHE); the University of California, San Francisco, Pediatric Environmental Health Specialty Unit (UCSF PEHSU); the Office of Environmental Health Hazard Assessment, California EPA (OEHHA); and the Science and Environmental Health Network (SEHN). Free continuing education credits are offered by the CDC and ATSDR to health professionals who complete stories presented in this e-book. *The Story of Health* is accessible from the CHE website at http://healthandenvironment. org/resources/story_of_health.

[Authors' note: It is an easy read and even has colorful pictures. Please don't be intimidated just because it offers credits to health professionals.]

Environmental Medicine Resources (Repeated from the Food Resource Guide)

American Academy of Environmental Medicine (AAEM)
The website of the AAEM can help you locate a doctor in your area who practices environmental medicine. They also have posted—on their website under "Quick Links"—their position statements, which provide an overview of their organization's philosophy. In particular, a paper titled "An Overview of Environmental Medicine" written by Gary R. Oberg, MD, FAAEM, explains the basics of environmental medicine and how its unique approach may provide additional help and answers to many suffering from chronic health problems. This paper was written with healthcare providers in mind, but is easy to read and understand. It can be accessed online at www. aaemonline.org.

Environmental Medicine Related Books by Doris J. Rapp, MD (Repeated from the Food Resource Guide):
- Is This Your Child?
- Is This Your Child's World?
- Our Toxic World: A Wake Up Call
- 32 Tips That Could Save Your Life

Doris J. Rapp, MD, is a board-certified environmental medical specialist and pediatric allergist and a *New York Times* best-selling author. Her first book, *Is This Your Child?*, describes the impact of food on children's behavior as well as their GI health. It helps parents identify common foods, chemicals, and allergic substances that could be causing behavior problems or your child to be sick or feel unwell. This book includes mini case studies describing various health problems encountered by children and adults, and the various environmental exposures that ended up being the root cause. The book *Our Toxic World: A Wake Up Call* discusses many chemical insults impacting our children's health (including food) and discusses ways you can prevent them. And her latest book, *32 Tips That Could Save Your Life,* may help you figure out exactly what it is that is making you sick, so you can better address the problem. More information on environmental factors affecting the health of both children and adults is available on the author's website at www. drrapp.com.

Resources for Chapter 9: Politics

Organizations Following Legislation
In each of the previous Resource Guide sections, we have listed many organizations involved in making positive changes and reforms in our food, environment, pharmaceuticals, and other consumer products. Most organizations follow any legislation in progress that will impact their particular area of interest and will keep members up-to-date about what is going on in the political arena, providing easy ways to help impact legislation. You can be just a click away from making a difference for our children. Check out the many, many consumer advocacy organizations we have listed in each of our previous Resource Guide sections if you want an opportunity to get involved in political changes. Great places to start include the Center for Food Safety, the Environmental Working Group, and Safer Chemicals, Healthy Families.

Safer Chemicals, Healthy Families Take Action
The Safer Chemicals, Healthy Families coalition represents more than 11 million individuals and over 450 organizations and businesses from across the nation, all united by their common concern about toxic chemicals in our homes, places of work, and everyday products. Visit the Safer Chemicals, Healthy Families website for more information on protecting our families from toxic chemicals and ways you can use your buying power to influence retailers and make a difference through their Mind the Store campaign. This campaign is making a real difference by pressuring businesses to remove toxic ingredients from our consumer products. Please visit Safer Chemicals, Healthy Families at www.saferchemicals.org for ways you can take action.

EWG's Take Action
Learn about action you can take right now regarding current legislation concerning chemicals in our food, water, and personal care products, as well as genetically modified foods, and farming pesticides by visiting the EWG's Action page at www.ewg.org/take-action.

Video Resource: *Citizens United v. FEC* (Federal Election Commission)
The Story of Stuff Project is a highly recommended and highly acclaimed online tool for learning more about environmental and consumer issues through web films made by creator and author Annie Leonard. Included in the series is a short video *The Story of Citizens United v. FEC*. It is a powerful movie that exposes the massive power that corporations exercise in our democracy. According to the Story of Stuff website, "The movie explores the history of American corporations and their political spending as well as the appropriate roles of citizens and for-profit corporations in our democracy. It demonstrates the far-reaching and toxic impact the Citizens United Supreme Court decision is having on our political process. It ends with a call to amend the U.S. Constitution to confirm that 'people' not corporations make the decisions in a democracy." You can view this short film and others on the Story of Stuff Project website under the Resources tab at www.storyofstuff.org.

Political Groups and Organizations
Below are just a few political (watchdog type) organizations you may want to check out that are working to protect our democracy and restore balance in our political system. They are concerned with the money, power, and influence large corporations are exerting in the political arena. We provided some website information from each organization to give you an idea about what they stand for.

The Center for Media and Democracy (CMD)

According to their website, "The Center for Media and Democracy is a national watchdog group that conducts in-depth investigations into corruption and the undue influence of corporations on media and democracy. CMD focuses on documenting key facts and revealing the impact of policies on ordinary people, not on what some PR spokesperson claims is true. With the cuts to newsrooms across the country, CMD's original and in-depth investigations are more important than ever in breaking through the spin of corporate-backed PR." Explore the CMD website at www.prwatch.org/cmd.

CMD also publishes SourceWatch to track corporations. SourceWatch provides well-documented information about corporate public relations (PR) campaigns including corporate front groups, people who "front" corporate campaigns, and PR operations. Check out the SourceWatch website at www.sourcewatch.org.

The Center for Responsive Politics

According to their website, "The Center for Responsive Politics is the nation's premier research group tracking money in U.S. politics and its effect of money on elections and public policy." They are a nonpartisan, independent, and nonprofit organization whose vision "is for Americans, empowered by access to clear and unbiased information about money's role in politics and policy, to use that knowledge to strengthen our democracy." They pursue their mission largely through their award-winning website, OpenSecrets.org, which is "the most comprehensive resource for federal campaign contributions, lobbying data and analysis available anywhere." Check out the Center for Responsive Politics website at www.opensecrets.org.

Move to Amend

According to the Move to Amend website, "Formed in September 2009, Move to Amend is a coalition of hundreds of organizations and hundreds of thousands of individuals committed to social and economic justice, ending corporate rule, and building a vibrant democracy that is genuinely accountable to the people, not corporate interests. We are calling for an amendment to the U.S. Constitution to unequivocally state that inalienable rights belong to human beings only, and that money is not a form of protected free speech under the First Amendment and can be regulated in political campaigns." Explore the Move to Amend website at www.movetoamend.org.

Public Citizen

According to their website, "Public Citizen serves as the people's voice in the nation's capital. Since its founding in 1971, Public Citizen has delved into an array of areas, but its work on each issue shares an overreaching goal: to ensure that all citizens are represented in the halls of power. For four decades, this organization has proudly championed citizen interests before Congress, the executive branch agencies, and the courts. It has successfully challenged the abusive practices of the pharmaceutical, nuclear, and automobile industries, and many others. Public Citizen is leading the charge against undemocratic trade agreements that advance the interests of mega-corporations at the expense of citizens worldwide." For more about Public Citizen, visit its website at www. citizen.org.

ABOUT THE AUTHORS

Joanne Stanton has a Bachelor of Science degree in Public Health from Temple University. She has fifteen years of experience working in the pharmaceutical industry as both a senior scientific communications writer and senior regulatory medical writer. Joanne also spent fifteen years coaching both high school and college field hockey and served briefly as the Associate Director of Athletics at Gwynedd-Mercy University. She lives in the Philadelphia area with her husband Marty. She has three sons and presently works as a self-employed medical writer in the pharmaceutical industry. She has also worked in the community in various volunteer positions including five years with the American Cancer Society's Childhood Cancer Program and Coaches vs. Cancer School Initiative Program. She is currently involved in community and political activism surrounding children's environmental health issues. Joanne believes that all paths following her son's brain tumor diagnosis have led her to research, write, and speak on the important messages contained in *Behind Closed Doors*.

Christine O'Donnell has a Bachelor of Science degree in Social Work from West Chester University. Christine worked as a social worker assisting the geriatric population and their families before starting a family of her own. Christine lives in the Philadelphia area with her husband John and four children. She is involved in environmental and political activism in her community as well as various other community-building projects and volunteer work including spearheading two recycling programs. Christine is an environmental enthusiast and natural advocate for children's health issues. The inspiration to create *Behind Closed Doors* originated after Christine's daughter suffered chronic health problems as an infant and toddler.

You can stay in touch with the authors and up to date about how you can best protect your children's health at www.behindcloseddoorsthebook.com.

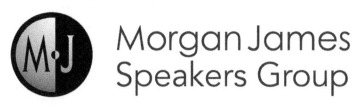

Morgan James
Speakers Group

We connect Morgan James published authors with live and online events and audiences who will benefit from their expertise.

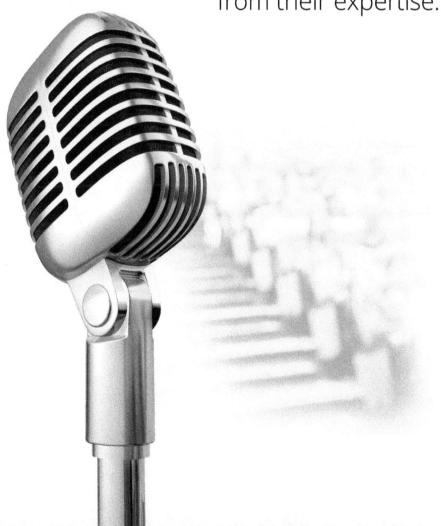

Printed in the USA
CPSIA information can be obtained
at www.ICGtesting.com
JSHW022213140824
68134JS00018B/1029